WHERE IT HURTS
AND WHY
HOW TO GAIN CONTROL
OF YOUR PAIN

Angela Sehgal, Ed.D., A.T.C./L.
and Kim Ortloff, L.M.T.

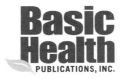

Basic
Health
PUBLICATIONS, INC.

The information contained in this book is based upon the research and personal and professional experiences of the authors. It is not intended as a substitute for consulting with your physician or other healthcare provider. Any attempt to diagnose and treat an illness should be done under the direction of a healthcare professional.

The publisher does not advocate the use of any particular healthcare protocol but believes the information in this book should be available to the public. The publisher and authors are not responsible for any adverse effects or consequences resulting from the use of the suggestions, preparations, or procedures discussed in this book. Should the reader have any questions concerning the appropriateness of any procedures or preparation mentioned, the authors and the publisher strongly suggest consulting a professional healthcare advisor.

Basic Health Publications, Inc.
8200 Boulevard East
North Bergen, NJ 07047
1-201-868-8336

Library of Congress Cataloging-in-Publication Data

Sehgal, Angela
    Where it hurts and why : how to gain control of your pain / Angela
Sehgal and Kim Ortloff.
        p. cm.
    Includes bibliographical references and index.
    ISBN 1-59120-065-2
    1. Pain—Popular works. 2. Pain—Treatment—Popular works.
I. Ortloff, Kim. II. Title.

    RB127.S396   2004
    616'.0472—dc22

                                                    2004008582

Editor: John Anderson
Illustrators: Jim Higdon and Chuck McCann
Typesetting/Book design: Gary A. Rosenberg
Cover design: Mike Stromberg

Printed in the United States of America

10   9   8   7   6   5   4   3   2   1

Contents

*I would like to dedicate this book
to the Lord who blesses me every day
and to my family and friends,
who support me as I strive to become complete.
This book is also dedicated to those people
who are seeking a better quality of life and health.
Persist, believe, understand, and act.*

—Angela Sehgal

*For my loving husband, John,
my biggest fan and supporter,
and best friend.*

—Kim Ortloff

Acknowledgments

I would like to acknowledge the following individuals who made the production of this book possible: my parents, brother, family, friends, colleagues, and students.

I would especially like to recognize my coauthor, Kim Ortloff, for her vision, energy, and will. Thank you for sharing this journey with me. You give great hugs! I look forward to another trip to New York!

To Jim Higdon, thank you for the endless hours of drawing. We can help you with your carpal tunnel syndrome! You have illustrated the human body beautifully.

To Chuck McCann, thank you for your willingness to rescue us in the eleventh hour. You, too, are a very talented artist.

To Dr. Barbara Mann, my professor, mentor, and friend, thank you for your words of wisdom and support.

Finally, a sincere thank you goes to our publisher, Norman Goldfind, who believed in this project and has supported our effort to share the word about feeling better fast and improving the quality of people's lives.

—Angela Sehgal

First and foremost, I would like to thank God for blessing me with the opportunity to express my passion in life with everyone. For it is through Him that I shine.

A very special thanks to my parents, Victor and Judi. Thank you for showing me the world and always letting my light shine. Your encouragement, guidance, discipline, and love taught me that we can have anything we want in life if we express our vision and create the reality. Accomplishing a goal is all about taking that first step and breaking through the seams of fear. It was your examples of leadership, love, and charisma that guided me. I love you both.

There are special people who are no longer with me but who have greatly influenced my philosophy of life. To my Nana and Popaw Vandenberg: their unselfishness and love provided a great example for me. They were always willing to help anyone, no matter the circumstances.

I would also like to thank Nana and Popaw Finnegan, Frank and Ken, and all my other family members, close friends, and clients (you know who you are) for their support, encouragement, and belief in me. You have provided endless efforts to support my goals and always took the extra step when something needed to get done. For all my clients, thank you for "doing your homework" and making improvements to your own health. It is not I who have helped you, but you who have stepped forward to help yourselves with knowledge and enthusiasm. Take your newly found knowledge and spread it to others. May we continue to laugh, smile, and hug! Keep stretching!

A special thanks to my mentor and great friend, Aaron Mattes. You have opened your heart to me and willingly shared your knowledge to further my education in physical rehabilitation and as a person. A great leader is one who helps to create leaders, who sees tremendous potential in a person and provides support and encouragement to help them achieve their goals. Aaron, you have always believed in me and shown me that quality of leadership. For that, I am very grateful and honored to promote your years of hard work, love, and knowledge—and to help spread it throughout the world. God bless you and your family.

To Angela, my coauthor, who looked at me in amazement and shock when I suggested that we needed to take a trip to New York to get this book published. (Angela was right in the middle of defending her dissertation.) You have incredible belief in me and took a leap of faith at my suggestion. All I can say is you better buckle up and get ready!

A special thanks to our illustrator, Jim Higdon, for your patience, incredible talent, and all the hours spent away from your family. I am grateful you agreed to join our team. And a special thanks to Jim's family for allowing us to take him away from them.

And finally, Chuck, thank you for saving us at the end of our journey!

—Kim Ortloff

Foreword

Pain can be an all-consuming problem: it may limit your ability to work, exercise, travel, and enjoy your leisure moments. Computers, couches, and reclining chairs contribute to poor posture and pain. Sitting places eight times more pressure on the lower back than standing. The leading cause of pain is ischemia, which is a lack of oxygen supply to the muscles, fasciae, and nerves. A buildup of toxins in the cells and failure of the lymphatic system contribute greatly to sickness, pain, and eventually death.

Where It Hurts and Why is a long overdue inspirational and motivational guide to self-evaluation and better living. It provides a rich supply of information to help restore optimum physiologic functioning of neural, lymphatic, and vascular systems, as well as our body's biochemical, biomechanical, and piezoelectric (biocurrent) homeostasis. Most important of all, we should understand that this book mirrors the very lives of these authors.

Physicians, chiropractors, osteopaths, physical therapists, exercise physiologists, massage therapists, trainers, coaches, and athletes, as well as anyone concerned about wellness and health, will find this book informative and effective for postural restoration, performance enhancement, injury prevention, and rehabilitation.

—Aaron L. Mattes, M.S., R.K.T., L.M.T.

Introduction

"When I was growing up, my mother always said life begins at forty," recalls Evelyn. "I always found it a strange saying because at age forty, I had already had six surgeries for endometriosis and then a total hysterectomy." In the days following her surgery, Evelyn began to have a burning feeling all over her body. She says it felt "as though I'd been exposed to freezing weather, where your face burns and feels cold and hurts all at the same time." Her body would at times be stiff from the pain.

This was the beginning of Evelyn's long journey to find the answer to what was going on in her body, a search that took her from Tallahassee, Florida, to the Mayo Clinic in Jacksonville, and on to Atlanta and Philadelphia. She was willing to try anything or go anywhere to find relief from her pain; however, none of the medicines that were prescribed helped. "I told one doctor that the medicine wasn't working and he told me to just take more," she recalls. "One day shortly after that, I woke up and couldn't move. I just lay there and cried. I didn't want to live on drugs—I wanted my life back. When I was finally able to get up, I flushed all the medicine down the toilet and started yet another search."

One day, Evelyn, stiff and barely able to walk, ran into a friend. Her friend had an appointment to see me (Kim) in an hour, but she had Evelyn take her place. On her first visit, she had very limited range of motion in her legs. After years of living in pain from her gynecological problems and the burning sensations, Evelyn's body kept holding on to the pain. As Evelyn said, "I see it as a peanut-butter-and-jelly sandwich: the muscles are the bread and the pain is the chunky peanut butter getting stuck between the muscles."

As I worked with Evelyn, we went through layer by layer, releasing the pain. I taught Evelyn step-by-step how to stretch and why stretching is important to help rid her body of pain. She was ischemic and the stretching exercises promoted blood flow, which enhanced the healing process of the muscles. Stretching also took the tension out of the tissue and allowed the muscle to move more freely with less stress on the joints. I developed stretching and strengthening protocols for her to do at home regularly and while traveling for her job.

I also emphasized the importance of proper diet and exercise and offered motivation and encouragement. After the first session, Evelyn walked out of the office pain-free, which inspired her to do her homework. Over the next year, her range of motion greatly improved, her pain was reduced by 95 percent, and her diet was much healthier. She now exercises daily and has lost over thirty pounds. By changing her diet, she has been able to control the burning feeling as well. Evelyn also started acupuncture, which has been another effective therapy for reducing her pain.

Evelyn is a new person with a new outlook on life. "It's a journey—sometimes one has to take control of one's own health and seek out alternatives," Evelyn reflects. "I still don't have all the answers, but I feel you have to take action in overseeing your health rather than live on medications for life."

THE PAINFUL TRUTH

Pain is the number-one reason for doctor visits. If you live with pain, you are not alone—it is estimated that 100 million Americans live with chronic pain. This number does not include the millions of people who experience acute pain from injuries every year. Pain can be caused by a variety of sources, including mental and emotional stress, poor posture, repetitive stress injuries from work, accidents, muscle strains from exercise, as a side effect of another illness (arthritis, migraines), and, as Evelyn discovered, as a lingering problem due to surgery. Sometimes the cause of pain is unknown.

It is estimated that headaches, back pain, arthritis, muscle aches, and joint pain lead to over $60 billion in lost productivity and missed workdays every year. And while conventional therapies such as medications can provide temporary relief, they often fail to address the root cause of pain. As you'll see, much of this suffering and expense is unnecessary.

Pain is a very subjective experience—each person perceives his or her own pain differently. How pain affects a person is influenced by their emotional and mental attitudes, earlier experiences with pain, other health conditions, and even spiritual beliefs. Often, both physiological and psychological factors must be addressed to alleviate pain. We believe that it is vital for the person suffering with some form of pain to understand its causes and take an active role in his or her own therapy.

THE JOURNEY TO BETTER HEALTH

Do you have to live in constant pain? No, you have a choice and a role in your recovery and healing. In this book, we will guide you on a journey to understanding pain and achieving better health using these action steps:

- Gain a better awareness of yourself (mind, body, and soul)

- Take charge of your health care and become proactive in your recovery

- Become motivated and inspired to achieve a better quality of life, regardless of your condition

Where It Hurts and Why illustrates these important aspects of wellness and health through easy-to-understand text and user-friendly anatomical diagrams. The diagrams will help you locate areas of discomfort, while text and illustrations will help you implement self-help techniques to ease your pain—stretching, strengthening exercises, and massage. You will also discover the profound importance of a positive mental attitude, a healthy lifestyle, and sound nutrition. Inspirational true stories—the stories of our own clients—and humor highlight the action steps included in this book. Our goal is to help you increase your awareness of your own body, boost your self-esteem, and encourage you to take control.

In Chapter 1, we discuss the physiology of pain and explore why the body hurts. The first step in healing is to gain a better awareness of yourself and what is causing your pain. Physical, mental, and emotional stresses can all contribute to pain; a worksheet is included to help identify these factors in your life.

Chapter 2 looks at how to manage the underlying causes of your pain. Eliminating pain means creating a healthier lifestyle. A positive attitude can greatly alleviate your pain and lead to a quicker recovery. Other actions you can take include eating a healthy diet, getting enough sleep, removing stressors from your environment, and finding humor and inspiration in your life.

In Chapter 3, we'll show you the action steps you can take now for pain relief. A number of simple strategies have proven remarkably effective in relieving aches and pains, including stretching, strengthening exercises, and massage techniques. The chapter also has instructions for immediate treatment of acute pain.

Chapters 4–9 provide detailed recommendations—specific stretches, exercises, and massage techniques—for pain in different areas of the body:

- Neck and shoulder

- Torso

- Arm, wrist, and hand

- Hip and low back

- Knee and upper leg

- Lower leg, ankle, and foot

Finally, Chapter 10 provides advice on when to seek professional help if your pain doesn't go away. We'll explore topics such as what questions to ask the doctor and how to avoid being put off by your doctor so that you can get the information you need.

Where It Hurts and Why can help guide you to a better quality of life: active, healthy, and free of pain. By combining the sports medicine fields of athletic training and massage therapy in an inspirational, humorous, and motivational way, we hope to assist and facilitate your healing and well-being.

Chapter 1

Why the Body Hurts

The body never lies.

—MARTHA GRAHAM (1894–1991)

As the crowd roared, there was an electric vibration in the air—it was a beautiful afternoon for a college soccer game. The score was tied and there were only a few minutes left in the game. Suddenly, one of the players from the home team stole the ball, broke away from the other players, and quickly moved up the field toward the goal. Janet, the goalie, was left alone to defend against the oncoming player's shot on goal. Janet quickly reacted and lunged toward the player in hopes of preventing the game-winning score.

In the attempt to block the shot, Janet collided with the other player and dropped to the ground in excruciating pain. The coach and athletic trainer rushed onto the field as Janet clutched her lower leg. A silence immediately fell over the crowd as it became obvious that her injury was very serious. As the ambulance transported Janet to the nearest hospital, it was whispered through the crowd that she had severely fractured her tibia, one of the bones in her lower leg.

The orthopedic surgeons at the hospital repaired the broken tibia by placing a metal rod in the middle of the bone to support the fracture site. Janet was then placed in a recovery room where she would stay for the next several days. The day following surgery, she experienced labored breathing, and diagnostic tests revealed that she had developed a blood clot in her lung.

This complication was only the beginning of Janet's long struggle to overcome what was perceived as a routine surgical repair. During the next several months, Janet would suffer from blood clots in her lungs, mononucleosis, and repeated surgeries to cleanse wound infections due to incisions and stitches. Janet's body began to reject the first metal rod, thus requiring several subsequent surgeries.

Janet's injury serves as an example of pain. Even if you have not suffered a severe injury similar to Janet's, you have no doubt experienced pain to some degree—back pain, headaches, muscle strains, athletic injuries, fractures, and so on. While pain is a natural mechanism the body uses to protect itself, it can also become a debilitating, chronic problem that interferes with daily life.

As you will learn in this chapter, there are different kinds of pain that can be caused by a variety of factors. While injuries such as Janet's are the most straightforward cause of pain, other factors such as stress or emotional upsets can also play a role. Not only that, but the actual experience of pain varies from individual to individual. We'll explore these topics, and then we'll help you discover what is causing your pain.

WHAT IS PAIN?

Pain can be defined as an uncomfortable sensation that indicates something is wrong. You could think of pain as a flashing signal that is alerting you to a problem. Those flashing pain signals can range from mild to moderate to severe. The signals travel via nerves throughout the body that communicate with the brain.

Your body has a complex network of communication lines (nerves) that transmit pain signals to and from the brain. This network serves as protection against injury and illness. For example, let's say you stubbed your toe. The injury message is immediately sent to your brain, which serves as an emergency communication cen-

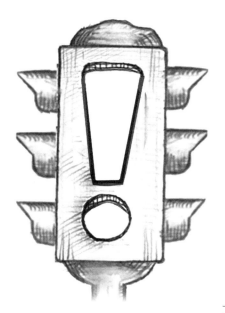

ter for the body. In turn, the brain sends out a pain message that something is wrong and dispatches a rescue team to the injured area. In the case of a minor injury or illness, the rescue team may be made up of microscopic cells. These microscopic cells respond much like a clean-up crew would after a wild party. They repair damaged areas with collagen and other reparative materials and chemicals as well as clean up the trauma site by absorbing cellular debris to allow for an increase of blood flow in the damaged area. In a severe case, there may be the need for a human rescue team, such as paramedics.

Think of pain as a flashing signal that is alerting you to a problem.

The brain sends out a pain message that something is wrong and dispatches a rescue team to the injured area.

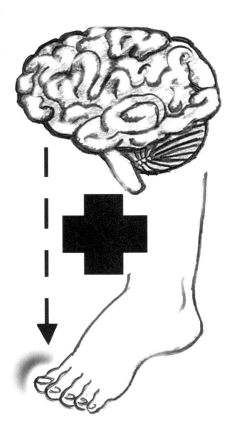

Paying attention to your body's pain signals is vital to improving your quality of life. The pain messages you experience should serve as a motivator for you to take action; pain is not something you should live with, work through, ignore, or avoid.

There are two basic types of pain: acute and chronic. Acute pain is like a sudden burst or explosion of sensation, stemming from an injury such as a sprained ankle or a stubbed toe. It happens quickly and causes severe or sharp pain that usually dissipates (resolves) in a short period of time. Acute pain resolves faster than chronic pain because the inflammation-and-pain cycle elapses much more quickly and without complications. On the other hand, chronic pain, such as arthritis, is like uninvited company: it hangs around for a long time and sometimes never goes away. Chronic pain lingers because of several factors, including severity of the injury or illness, inaccurate diagnosis, inadequate treatment, poor physical, mental, or emotional status, and a prolonged cycle of inflammation, pain, and spasm. It is estimated that over 100 million Americans suffer from chronic pain.

THE EXPERIENCE OF PAIN

Pain is a very natural process and we all experience it. However, everyone feels pain differently. The way the brain interprets pain determines how we react to varying levels of pain. Tolerance levels will vary from person to person depending on a number of stressors placed on the body—diet, emotional stress, drugs, poor attitude, and so on.

For example, I (Kim) recently worked with a sixty-year-old man, Don, who has severely arthritic knees. His doctors have been after him for several years to get

Referred and Radiating Pain

Referred pain is pain felt somewhere other than the source area. For example, pain felt in the left shoulder (if you've had no previous injury) may be the signal of a heart attack, or it may be due to acid reflux disease or a hiatal hernia. The true source of referred pain can be very difficult to figure out. *Radiating pain* is pain that is felt from the source and all along the route of a nerve. A common example of this is sciatic pain, which is felt from the low back, through the buttocks, and down the back of the leg (along the sciatic nerve).

For diagnosis and evaluation of referred or radiating pain, it is important to consult a healthcare professional. If you are suffering from either of these types of pain, you could have a serious medical condition that should be treated immediately by your physician. In some cases, referred or radiating pain could be a sign of a life-threatening illness.

knee-replacement surgery. He walks with a cane and suffers daily from pain. His pain used to be bad enough that he would sometimes slide down the stairs on his backside instead of stepping down. Don began working extensively with a flexibility-and-strengthening program, chiropractic care, and acupuncture. As a result, he lessened his pain by over 80 percent, convincing him to wait as long as medically possible before having surgery (if at all). His experience triggered his enthusiasm to make a difference and feel better. "Life is too short to hurt and I now realize I am in control," says Don. His pain is now manageable because he felt empowered with a positive outlook and took the steps necessary to improve his diet and exercise regimen.

In other words, your experience of pain can be positively affected by taking a proactive approach to changing your life for the better. Many people who simply rely on anti-inflammatory medications and narcotics to relieve or eliminate their pain typically refuse to take a proactive stance and end up staying in pain much longer. Others like Don are willing to embrace a proactive approach first: Don stayed away from narcotics and instead used "hands-on" therapies to help himself through proper nutrition and exercise.

"Pain is what the patient says it is," states Scott Fishman, M.D., in his book *The War on Pain.* "Personal psychology and physiology—the mind and the body—mingle to shape the exact outline of your experience with pain. Like personality, your pain tolerance is a product of personal biology as well as memories, experiences, behavior patterns, family history, and culture." Often as children, we monitored our parents' behavior, so a reaction to pain displayed by a parent may help mold the child's reaction to pain. For example, imagine a parent stepping on a sharp object while walking across the driveway: if the parent reacts by taking a deep breath and laughing their way through the discomfort, then the child perhaps learns that discomfort can be a humorous experience versus a painful one.

Through our experiences in sports medicine, we have recognized differences in pain tolerance among athletes. Anecdotally, female athletes tend to endure pain at a much higher level than male athletes, and older collegiate athletes seem to possess better pain-coping strategies than younger athletes. Plus, athletes with prior pain experiences tend to recover with fewer complications than athletes with no previous pain experience. In other words, the athletes who have "been there, done that" already know what to expect in terms of treatment, rehabilitation, and recovery. These factors may contribute to quicker healing and recovery.

"The way we experience chronic pain is affected not merely by the physical processes that have caused it, but also by our intellectual and emotional reaction to it," according to Dr. Leon Chaitow in his book *Conquer Pain the Natural Way*. "Much depends on the 'meaning' that we give pain, which we tend to process through our individual experiences and expectations." For example, Ted was experiencing chest pain, rapid heart rate, and heavy breathing. Because he did not understand the root cause (meaning) of his chest pain and discomfort, he began to panic. Ted thought the worst—I'm dying of a heart attack—thus aggravating his symptoms. By attaching a different meaning to the problem—that he wasn't having a heart attack—he could shift his thinking and reduce his pain.

In Janet's case, on the other hand, her positive intellectual and emotional reaction to pain played a significant role in her recovery. Although she suffered a severe trauma, she kept an optimistic attitude and focused on her goal of returning to play collegiate soccer. By taking a proactive approach to therapy, Janet did not let her pain get in the way of her recovery.

Do you have to suffer with chronic pain? No! According to Bernie Siegel, M.D., in his book *Love, Medicine, and Miracles,* "We must pay attention to our feelings and let them guide us. If you ignore your body and messages, there will be consequences." The key to a better quality of life is in understanding pain and its purpose; then take active steps to alleviate it.

CAUSES OF PAIN

By identifying specific types and regions of pain, you can become more proactive in managing your discomfort, identifying the source, and possibly eliminating the root cause of your pain.

What is causing your pain? Choose from the following list or fill in your own answer in the space provided.

- ❏ Injury, direct trauma
- ❏ Repetitive stress/excessive motion (computer work, typing)
- ❏ Accident(s)
- ❏ Poor posture
- ❏ Disease
- ❏ Surgery
- ❏ Exercise
- ❏ Stress
- ❏ Unknown cause
- ❏ Other _____

Stress is often overlooked as a source of pain, as Anika found out. Anika, an exercise enthusiast, could sense that something was seriously wrong with her health. One morning as she was driving to the gym, her skin suddenly felt clammy and started to tingle. "At that moment, I thought my heart was going to pop out of my chest due to palpitations," Anika said. "I was very scared driving that morning. As someone who is in shape, I took my health for granted." Anika thought that if she looked good on the outside, everything would be fine on the inside of her body. That particular morning, Anika felt that something was clearly wrong with her normal state of health and took action. It was that experience that inspired her to seek professional help.

Anika typifies a large number of people who believe they are "healthy" when in fact they are not. Some people do not know the difference between being healthy or unhealthy. Luckily, Anika paid attention to the warning signals and immediately sought medical help. According to Anika, "It is difficult being a patient when you are seemingly so healthy." With guidance from her physician, Anika began researching her symptoms through books and the Internet. "I never really understood what happened that day until I started doing research on my condition. With the help of my doctor, I discovered that although my symptoms were physical, the triggers could have been mental or emotional. That discovery amazed me!" The doctor's diagnosis of a stress disorder caused Anika to stop what she was doing and attend to her pain signals.

"It's often said that stress is one of the most destructive elements in people's daily lives, but that's only a half truth," says Dr. Siegel in *Love, Medicine, and Miracles.* "The way we react to stress appears to be more important than stress itself." Pain itself causes stress, which can cause the cycle of inflammation, pain, and spasm to increase in severity. On the other hand, if you decrease stress, you can break the cycle, leading to faster pain relief.

Does Anika's, Janet's, or Ted's story of pain relate to you? We have all felt pain, but have we taken the time to recognize the root cause of our pain or stress? Listed in Table 1.1 are more examples of possible sources of pain—physical, emotional, and mental. Which sources are affecting you? Fill in the blanks with your own words, if you like.

TABLE 1.1. POSSIBLE PAIN-CAUSING STRESSORS

PHYSICAL	EMOTIONAL	MENTAL
Poor posture	Divorce	Time pressures
Injury/trauma	Death of family member/friend	Anxiety/depression
Yard work	Loss of job	Burnout
Fitness program	Work environment	Setting high goals
Losing/gaining weight	Relationships	Perfectionist/worrywart
Childbirth	Financial stress	Too many commitments
Other:	*Other:*	*Other:*

WHAT IS A PAIN SCALE?

Pain scales are used to help quantify and give standardized values to a patient's level of pain. They assist healthcare professionals in measuring the patient's progress, whether it is positive or negative. Generally, the level of pain can be used as an indication of the severity of the problem. For example, if you register a "7" on the pain scale before stretching, strengthening, and treatment and afterward the pain has decreased to a "3," you have made progress in your recovery and healing. Obviously, this is a subjective judgment, but it still provides an initial assessment of pain level. What is your level of pain? Indicate it on the pain scale (see Figure 1.1).

Your Pain Worksheet

Figure 1.2 provides a unique pain worksheet to assist you in identifying and chart-

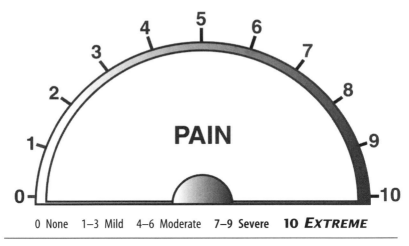

0 None   1–3 Mild   4–6 Moderate   7–9 Severe   **10** *EXTREME*

FIGURE 1.1. PAIN SCALE   (Indicate your level of pain by drawing an arrow.)

ing your pain. The pain worksheet serves as a visible tool for you to use during your journey to better health. You can use the pain worksheet to chart your progress and develop a plan of action from the items provided in each category. Remember that you must address your pain in all three realms, including the mind, body, and soul.

We recommend that you use this pain worksheet daily (make photocopies of page 13 before using). Follow these directions when completing the worksheet:

1. Complete the pain scale provided in the top left corner—indicate your numerical score by circling the appropriate number.

2. Indicate your "zones of pain" on the anatomical charts by placing an "X" over your painful area(s). Note that the corresponding chapter numbers are given on the left side of each zone.

3. Review the nutrition pyramid on the bottom left of the worksheet.

4. In the Day 1 column, indicate your pain level in the pain scale provided at the top. Use the same pain scale already provided.

5. Check the boxes that apply to your current status in the sections on mind, body, and soul.

6. Continue down the Day 1 column and develop your plan of action for mind, body, and soul.

7. Repeat steps 4–6 for Day 2 and subsequent days.

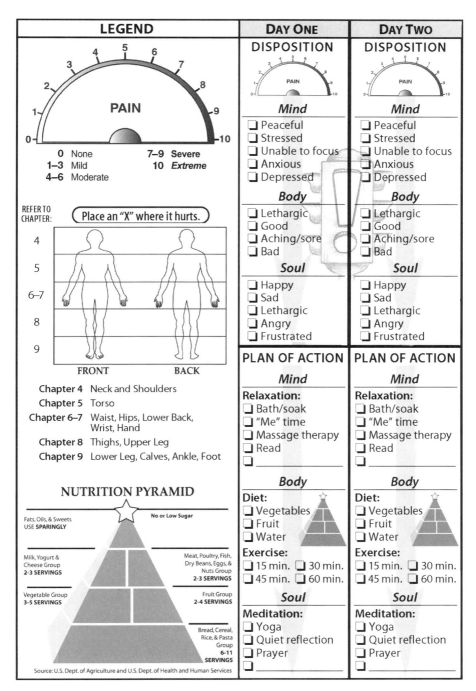

FIGURE 1.2. PAIN WORKSHEET (See instructions on page 12.)

On your worksheet, note the daily progress of your health and the level of pain on your pain scale. If you follow the action steps provided in the following chapters, you should begin to feel a difference in your health. If not, take this worksheet to your professional healthcare provider and discuss other action steps that might meet your needs.

MORE ABOUT JANET

I (Kim) saw Janet twice weekly for several weeks. She learned the proper way to stretch and strengthen the badly injured area and how to apply self-massage techniques at home to further her therapy. All of these modalities combined helped her condition remarkably. Most important, she developed a new outlook for herself and her future. She continued to have complications and surgeries but always had her own therapy to fall back on, which assisted her recovery time. To date, Janet has undergone eight surgeries related to her tibial fracture. Even so, she has maintained a positive mental attitude throughout her healing process. This shows the importance of gaining control of your pain and involving yourself in getting better. Janet has permanent deformity of her lower leg and foot and some loss of function of her toes on the injured leg, but she continues to practice and play soccer at the collegiate level.

By learning more about your pain, taking charge of your treatment by using the therapeutic approaches outlined in this book, and tracking your progress with the pain worksheet, you too can adopt a proactive and positive attitude toward pain relief.

Chapter 2

How to Manage Your Pain: The Components of Complete Health

Now that you have seen the blueprint of pain, it is time to go to the next level of pain recognition: managing your pain through the components of complete health. Managing pain is similar to building a house. You start by laying the foundation (pouring the concrete) to create a very sound and solid structure. Once the foundation has cured, the frame of the house is constructed, which provides the internal skeleton for the walls and the roof. After the walls and roof have been completed, the details of the inside of the house are then worked on, producing, in the end, a finished product.

This chapter illustrates similar "building" techniques for alleviating your pain, teaching you how to incorporate the components of complete health into your life. Your building blocks are a positive mental attitude (the foundation) to motivate you, healthy habits (walls and roof) to create a healthier body and environment, and the ability to incorporate these elements of better health into everyday life (the finished product). You will then be ready to move into your new pain-free body!

A POSITIVE MENTAL ATTITUDE (THE FOUNDATION)

Your attitude today determines your success for tomorrow.

—KEITH HARRELL, FROM *ATTITUDE IS EVERYTHING*

Simply put, you achieve what you believe! The power of positive thinking is an investment: it compounds over time, leaving your heart rich, your soul abundant, and your life prosperous. Each of us has a choice in how we react to our own pain. In the pain experience, our reaction can range from positive to negative. In effect, our mind has control over our reaction. In a positive reaction to pain, a "challenge" is presented. At this point, a positive outlook helps to defeat the problem at hand, and our recovery time can be lessened. In a negative reaction, pain is considered a hindrance that is worsening our symptoms, thus elevating our fear, anger, and frustration—and lengthening our recovery.

The power of suggestion can play a significant role in our response to pain (for example, in the case of a simple paper cut). The brain blocks the pain out until the eyes recognize the injury, a connection which then feeds the brain numerous signals. As we learned earlier, the brain is the 911 emergency center of the body—once alerted, it sends for help (the rescue team). By feeding kinder thoughts to our emergency center, the pain reaction may be minimized. On the flip side, a negative reaction could worsen the symptoms, thus creating a more painful experience. According to Kris Stowers, M.D., of the Tallahassee Orthopedic Clinic, in Florida, "One of the most critical aspects to dealing with injuries is a positive attitude, which not only increases effort and motivation but also helps deal with the pain of injury and pain during rehabilitation." Try talking kindly to yourself (a positive pep talk) the next time you cut your finger or stub your toe—saying or thinking words or phrases that encourage or motivate you in a constructive manner.

Learn to Be Positive

A new positive attitude leads to a much healthier life, a renewed sense of well-being, and increased confidence. You may think this is a difficult task, but don't get discouraged—there are numerous ways to help change your thinking from negative to positive.

Surrounding yourself with positive people or people you admire is a great place to start. Establish a new Rolodex of people who share positive beliefs, goals, and attitudes. Successful people, of all walks of life, are typically willing to share their expe-

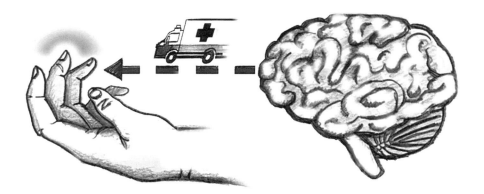

The brain is the 911 emergency center of the body—once alerted, it sends for help (the rescue team).

Stephanie's Story

Stephanie shares the story of her childbirth experience. Shortly before going into labor with her first child, Stephanie had an appointment with her doctor. The doctor's conversation with her transpired as follows: "Stephanie, I want you to have a positive and healthy birthing experience without the use of pain-relieving drugs. This will be healthier for you and the baby. Throughout my years in child delivery, we have avoided drugs through the use of a positive mind-set, motivation, enthusiasm, and support from family and friends. I'm offering all of the above and am here to support you through this entire natural process." Stephanie was so impressed by his positive and caring attitude. "You could really see the excitement and concern in his eyes. I felt comfortable instantly." Stephanie was very willing to make this first birthing experience a healthy one. She focused on maintaining a positive attitude daily, at the doctor's suggestion. Stephanie experienced a healthy and exhilarating childbirth and followed the same natural protocol for the birth of her second child.

riences with anyone who will ask. They can inspire you with their stories and help you along on your journey toward better health and well-being.

For example, Mark Victor Hansen, author of *Chicken Soup for the Soul,* started out his career bankrupt. Instead of dwelling on the negative, and with the help of family and friends, he used his bankruptcy experience as an opportunity to inspire others with heart-warming and positive stories. *Chicken Soup for the Soul* has since sold over 50 million copies worldwide. Mark and his coauthor, Jack Canfield, also donated a percentage of their proceeds to several charities—giving back to those in need serves as a reminder of their difficult past.

Everyone will have his or her own starting point, and additional positive resources may be necessary for some individuals. Other helpful resources include networking or church groups, personal instruction in the form of counseling, the Internet, reading materials, and motivational tapes or CDs. All of these resources are readily available, even if you do not have a lot of money. Keith Harrell's book *Attitude Is Everything* offers a valuable series of steps for building a more positive outlook. Among these steps, you may find the starting point you need. For instance, Harrell suggests reframing your bad attitude by avoiding negative words such as *can't, won't,* and *don't* and replacing them with positive words of action. Another step calls for seeing change as an opportunity and, thereby, altering your lifestyle to alleviate pain.

Joe's Story

Joe was diagnosed with Hodgkin's disease, which meant he had to undergo a "brutal" regimen of chemotherapy every month. In the early 1980s, there were not many good antinausea medicines available; nausea was the most common side effect of chemotherapy treatment. But Joe had a strong mind-over-matter philosophy. For his post-chemotherapy "attitude adjustment," he would go home, put on his running shoes, and take to the roads. Anyone who has ever experienced chemotherapy knows that this is no small feat. Most folks are in the bathroom with their heads close to the commode or they are flat on their backs in bed. His mental and physical strength and his attitude are the things that got him through the treatment and ultimately helped him overcome the disease. After several months of chemotherapy, Joe went into remission and is alive and healthy to this day.

Thought is the blossom; language the bud;
action the fruit behind it.
—Ralph Waldo Emerson

Setting Goals

The purpose of setting goals is to help clarify what you are looking for or what you want in life, including the financial, spiritual, physical, mental, emotional, professional, and personal realms of life. A goal is "the ongoing pursuit of a worthy objective until accomplished," according to Jack Canfield, Mark Victor Hansen, and Les Hewitt's book *The Power of Focus*. What does this sentence really mean? "*Ongoing* means it's a process, because goals take time. *Pursuit* indicates a chase may be involved. *Worthy* shows that the chase will be worthwhile, that there's a big enough reward at the end to endure the tough times. *Until accomplished* suggests you'll do whatever it takes to get the job done. Not always easy, but essential if you want a life full of outstanding accomplishments."

The first step is to take some time and think about what your goals might be. Perhaps the best way to get going is to write down your goals. Here are some suggestions to help you:

• You can never write too many goals; separate them into the categories mentioned above— financial, spiritual, physical, mental, emotional, professional, and personal.

- Your goals should be meaningful to you.

- Be specific with dates for completing each goal, time you want to spend on it, and other quantifiable aspects—this helps make your goal something more concrete.

- Use action words instead of nonaction words in writing your goals (nonaction words: *if only, I wish, what if;* action words: *I am so happy that, I will, I will not*).

- Be honest in setting your goals.

Feel free to share some of your goals with family or friends. They can help keep you on track and support you in achieving your goals. Think from your dreams and establish your desired end result. If you have imagined your end result, then the process becomes much clearer. Be specific! For example, if you want to lose weight, decide how many pounds you want to lose each week. If you want to run a marathon, set up a training schedule. Set your goals accordingly and find a support system.

Fun Challenge

Write down as many goals as you can. Express yourself freely and be as crazy as you want. Remember, this is about you, your dreams, wishes, and desires. Read your goals daily, in the morning preferably, and make them come true.

If you think you can or think you can't, you're right.

—HENRY FORD

Affirmations

Do not try to be optimistic, *become* optimistic. Affirmation can be defined as a declaration of a belief to uphold and confirm. Words alone can leave you empty, but if you develop your words into affirming positive statements, they can lead to acceptance, belief, and action. "Affirmations, when used with faith in their effectiveness, can bolster our determination to overcome the enslavement of pain," according to Dr. Leon Chaitow in his book *Conquer Pain the Natural Way*. Keep in mind that simplicity is the key to writing affirmations. Below are some examples of life affirmations:

- I feel great today.
- I feel rich, abundant, and prosperous.
- I am worthy of good things happening to me.
- I am smart and attractive.
- I love the way I look.
- My body feels healthy.

Fun Challenge

Write down your affirmations on three-by-five-inch index cards. Before going to bed at night, read these statements until you get sleepy. Remember, the subconscious mind never sleeps. As your eyes close, your brain may continue to wheel and deal with the day's events or perhaps you are still angry from an event that occurred a few days earlier. Get in the habit of training your mind to rest, slow down, and divert your energies to positive and thoughtful affirmations. Your affirmations may include statements such as:

- Tomorrow is going to be a great and prosperous day.

- I will feel healthy and happy.

- I will help as many people as I can.

- I will breathe deeply and keep feeding my subconscious mind with positive thoughts.

- I am thankful for what this day has brought.

Do Your Homework

Knowledge is power, especially when it comes to your own health. In the journey to improve all aspects of your life, including your health, getting a checkup may be the place to start. A thorough knowledge of your current state of health can help you prepare for the road ahead. Not many of us enjoy going to the doctor. Often, we feel inferior or scared. When visiting your doctor for an illness or injury, be prepared: write down all of your symptoms, use the pain worksheet in Chapter 1 to help track them, and ask questions. This will help your doctor gain a better understanding of you and your pain.

If and when a diagnosis has been made, educate and enlighten yourself on your condition. By "enlighten" we mean research your condition to increase your own awareness. Make it a priority in your schedule to investigate and learn more about your injury or medical condition. After all, you are the biggest stakeholder in your health and well-being.

Your research may require networking with other people or organizations that address your issues. Use your computer or library to search topics related to your situation. The Internet is a valuable place to find information—you have access to a huge amount of health and medical resources (see the Appendix for a list of pain-related websites). However, information on the Internet is not always vetted in the same way as books and medical journals, so it may be inaccurate. Also, because many websites are selling products or services, an attitude of healthy skepticism is advised.

Below are some guidelines to help you find reliable and accurate information.

- Do not rely on a single website.

- Make sure each website is up-to-date with the latest information.

- Research any online physician that you decide to consult. Your condition may warrant a face-to-face office visit. Use of online physicians may be valuable, but be aware of the positive and negative aspects of this type of health care; consider follow-up care, complications, referrals to specialists, and insurance coverage.

- Use common sense to avoid consumer-health fraud and always read the fine print.

- Keep all your personal information (social security number, address, phone number) confidential.

- Look for the HON seal of approval on websites: HON stands for Health on the Net Foundation; their goal is to separate what is reliable from what isn't.

- For more information on Internet sites related to health, see *Healthcare Online for Dummies* by Howard Wolinsky and Judi Wolinsky.

- Use a medical dictionary/encyclopedia and medical journals/literature as references.

- Know your own medicines and ask your physician and pharmacist questions.

- Contact national associations, such as the American Heart Association, the American Stroke Association, and the Muscular Dystrophy Association. National association websites are typically a very accurate source of information, and they continually update their medical information; refer to the Appendix for a list of these sites.)

- Become a member of support groups.

- Use audio support, such as CDs, related to your condition or illness.

- Locate a good hospital, which is a valuable resource for locating reliable medical professionals.

ESTABLISHING HEALTHY HABITS (WALLS AND ROOF)

If you want to have what you have not,
you must do what you have not done.

—Evan Esar

Now that we have poured our foundation with a positive attitude, it's time to begin the process of building the walls and the roof. If you thought the first section was challenging, get ready to create a healthier body and environment. Today, healthy habits are harder to maintain in our fast-paced society: many of us drive everywhere, eat fast food, and work long, stressful hours. In order to become healthy, we must practice healthy living—this means making yourself a priority by starting to exercise, achieving good nutrition, getting proper amounts of sleep, and reducing stress, thereby strengthening the mind, body, and soul.

Dedicate yourself to making these changes for improving your health and try to avoid temporary changes. For example, Sally started a new diet one week and was excited and energized by the prospect of improving her health. After the first week, however, the preparation of meals became a hassle and too time-consuming. As a result, Sally became frustrated, received no support from her husband, and finally gave up. If Sally had established a mindset to stick with her program, then set some nutritional goals and shared them with her husband, perhaps her outcome would have been different.

Cathie's Story

Life takes some unexpected turns, as Cathie found out. She was surprised when she was diagnosed with multiple sclerosis (MS), a disease of the nervous system and brain for which there is no cure. "How could this happen to me, a strong twenty-five-year-old runner?" she says. "I was attending a class in real estate when suddenly I could see out of only one eye. After an emergency appointment with an ophthalmologist and a subsequent appointment with a local neurologist, I was diagnosed with something that I did not understand—I had no idea what it was or how it was going to affect me." Cathie realized that she was lucky to have been diagnosed so quickly, since most people spend a long time "doctor shopping" before they know for sure that they have MS.

For years after the diagnosis, Cathie felt that she could deal with complications such as retro bulbar neuritis (inflammation of the optic nerve) and double vision, but she was starting to fall while running and this unnerved her. "I felt that I had to develop an action plan. Being a positive person, I thought I could handle this myself if I just ate right, rested, and moved my body."

Communicate your desires to anyone that can support or help you in any way. So many of us begin new habits and break them a week later because of frustration, time constraints, or lack of support from family and friends. Ask for help as you go through the transition of incorporating your new habits and action steps into daily living. Keep in mind that it takes twenty-one days to truly establish new habits. The key to healthy habits is good balance—avoid excess and have fun!

Fitness is imperative if we are to find ourselves,
win self respect, and meet life's challenges.

—JACK CANFIELD AND MARK VICTOR HANSEN,
FROM *DARE TO WIN*

Get Moving!

When beginning a new exercise program, take it slowly. Gradually start to move and become active, both indoors and outdoors, regardless of your physical condition. Why is exercise so important? It is estimated that as many as 250,000 Americans die

She tried the Swank low-fat diet for MS—it was quite a transition, but she stuck with it. She began to explore alternative therapies such as touch stimulation and methods to help stimulate new neural pathways within her neurological systems. Chiropractic care, body massage, Pilates classes, and stretching (with Kim) were all methods to encourage body parts affected by MS to work. "I began weight lifting to keep myself physically strong, prayer to keep myself centered, and counseling when needed. It's not just one item that helps me, but the combination that allows me to keep going."

Today, at fifty-four, she has resumed her childhood love of swimming, for aerobic workouts. She also walks for building her bones, lifts weights for strength, and does any activity her body can easily accomplish in a cool environment (overheating can exacerbate MS symptoms). "I have a philosophy that one has to keep moving and so I do." Cathie also takes several medications for her MS to help keep the illness from getting any worse.

"Emotionally, I have survived with the loving support of my husband, friends, and physicians, along with prayer. Multiple sclerosis is a disease that, no matter what I do or don't do, the course is unpredictable. At least I'm a healthier person for doing all I can."

each year due to an overly sedentary lifestyle. Plus, an active body is less likely to be debilitated by chronic pain.

It is never too late in life to start an exercise program and receive the health benefits of activity. However, not everyone enjoys going to the gym. And that's okay. You can get fit without long, sweaty workouts: studies have shown improvement in people's overall health when they simply choose to take the stairs instead of the elevator while at work, in shopping malls, and airports. Movement, in even its simplest form, is very beneficial for the health of the body.

If you are just starting to exercise, try dividing your workout time into manageable segments. Work out for ten minutes twice daily instead of once daily for twenty to thirty minutes. Try the 10,000-steps challenge, a recent innovation among healthcare professionals. Simply buy an inexpensive pedometer (a tool that counts your strides) and challenge yourself to take 10,000 steps per day. This includes walking stairs instead of taking elevators, sweeping the driveway, walking the dog, raking the yard, and so on. It's a perfect way to break up your exercise time.

Among its many benefits, exercise also:

- Reduces the risk and severity of medical problems

- Produces positive psychological benefits, such as increased confidence and self-esteem

- Decreases depression and stress, improves memory and mood

- Encourages better sleep patterns and cardiovascular function

- Promotes positive social benefits, such as increased family time (exercise together)

- Helps maintain ideal body weight

- Strengthens the immune system and increases metabolism and energy

- Decreases PMS (premenstrual syndrome) symptoms

- Improves balance, strength, flexibility, and posture; eases low-back pain

- Promotes a faster recovery time from injury or illness

- Reduces stress on bones, joints, ligaments, and the vascular system

- Works for everyone

Consider hiring a fitness professional to help you design an exercise program and keep you motivated. Most people quit after the first week, so set goals to inspire you and keep you motivated. Make changes as necessary to keep your interest, such as varying sports activities or weight-lifting routines. Find a workout buddy: having a support system helps improve your success rate, and it costs nothing to walk or run with a friend or family member.

If you're trying to lose weight, dieting plus exercise is the way to achieve the best results. "There is a reduction in metabolic rate (the rate at which the body burns energy) that occurs with dieting," according to Dr. Mike Overton, the department chair of the Nutrition, Food, and Exercise Sciences Department at Florida State University. "Exercise might help maintain weight loss during dieting."

Nutrition and Energy

All living creatures need food and water to survive. Your body is a living organism that fuels itself from what goes down the hatch. Food provides energy and nutrients, which help keep the body running. When your gas tank is low or empty, you will see a decline in different aspects of the body's function, including mental, physical, and emotional aspects.

During the digestive process, nutrients are extracted from the food we have consumed. Nutrients travel within the cellular tissues, along with blood and oxygen, and are sent throughout the body to areas that require tissue or bone repair. Nutrients are also essential for proper communications within the nervous system—and, thereby, are important for pain relief. This is why we stress a proper diet, consisting of the basic food groups.

Your body is composed of 60 percent water, 20 percent fat, and 20 percent protein, carbohydrates, and minerals. It is important to balance your diet to incorporate all of these components. Follow the guidelines of the USDA Food Guide Pyramid (see Figure 2.1) and remember that moderation is the key to success in nutrition and maintaining a normal weight. Avoiding extra weight can be important for alleviating some types of pain.

Generally, it's good to start out slowly and try to work in new habits gradually. First, cut food-portion sizes in half and learn to eat more slowly. The body takes more time digesting when food is chewed slowly and properly before it reaches the stomach, helping you feel satisfied sooner. And always eat breakfast! A protein shake, cottage cheese with fruit, or oatmeal and other cereals high in fiber are great examples. Avoid sugar and sugar substitutes.

Be careful with fast foods; eliminate them entirely if you can. Pack your lunch instead—it gives you control over what you eat and, in the long run, is much easier on the budget. Lunches can be as simple as fruit and half a sandwich. For snacks eat fruit that is high in fiber (such as apples and pears) instead of chips and crackers. Other good snack choices are dried fruit (apples, apricots, and so on) and nuts (eat the recommended single-portion size).

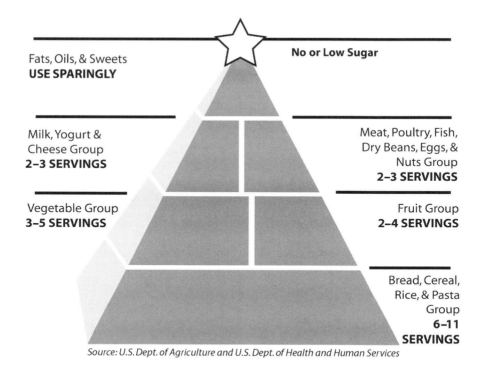

Source: U.S. Dept. of Agriculture and U.S. Dept. of Health and Human Services

FIGURE 2.1. USDA FOOD GUIDE PYRAMID

Legumes, lean meats, and fish are suitable for dinner, with a side salad and sweet potato. White potatoes, breads, and other heavy starches are considered simple sugars and can leave you feeling unsatisfied with possible sugar cravings. These foods are high on the glycemic food index: they are digested quickly and leave you feeling hungry. Stick to low glycemic foods, such as sweet potatoes, oatmeal, apples, oranges, lentils, brown rice, buckwheat pancakes, whole-wheat pasta, and whole-wheat bread. Avoid eating late dinners, as your metabolic rate naturally slows in the evening, which could lead to extra weight gain.

Stick to low-fat diets, but you shouldn't eliminate fat entirely. Avoid fat-free products, such as fat-free snack cakes, crackers, cookies, and so on, because high amounts of sugar may have been substituted to help develop the taste of these products. Read nutrition labels! Some nutrition labels on foods do not tell you the percent of fat per serving based on the caloric value; instead, they tell you the percentages based on the fat gram (fat is measured in weight). Your concern should be the percent of fat based on calories. One gram of fat equals 9 calories. Example: an energy bar contains 200 calories, with 6 grams of fat; the amount of fat calories is 54. Divide 54 into 200—this energy bar is 27 percent fat per serving! If you are trying to limit your diet to 15 percent fat, then this bar is not for you.

For healthier shopping, read ingredient lists on foods as well as nutrition labels. Look for whole ingredients. If the list is long, you probably don't want it—the fewer the ingredients, the more whole the food is. Eat as many organic foods as you can, especially produce. Low-fat cheeses, yogurt, and meats are good choices. Smart Balance Buttery Spread is a great choice over regular butter for its combination of healthy oils; olive oil is preferable to other vegetable oils. Cut out junk food and fake fats (partially hydrogenated or trans fats). Buy whole-wheat bread sticks instead of bran muffins and look for low sodium content in frozen diet foods and pizzas.

We always recommend a daily multivitamin and suggest you visit a nutritionist to get the proper supplementation for your individual constitution. Each person is different and may have different requirements. (Health food stores are typically pretty knowledgeable in this area also.) A nutritionist/dietician is a valuable asset, in addition to your physician—make one a part of your complete healthcare team.

Proper Hydration

In addition to your eating habits, consider the importance of proper water consumption. Not only is your body 60 percent water, but your muscles are actually 90 percent water. What does this mean? All of your soft tissues (muscle) and organs require a healthy quantity of water to function. Depletion of water can be very dangerous and cause dehydration, which is potentially fatal.

Your thirst mechanism is not a true indication of dehydration in your body. Unfortunately, we are not designed with an indicator needle that tells us when our water tanks are empty. So, it is important to drink water throughout the day, even when you do not feel thirsty. Consume eight to ten glasses a day. For variety, add lemon, orange, or lime juice to your water. If you're participating in athletic activities, you can lose about $1\frac{1}{2}$ quarts of body fluid per hour, so it is vital to reload your body with plenty of water.

What about drinking sports drinks or other fluids instead of water? Water is the best choice, or a combination of water and other fluids. Other fluids, such as coffee, teas, juices, commercial sports drinks, alcohol, and sodas (regular or diet), are not equal to water. Although these beverages provide water, some may also contain caffeine, high levels of sugar, and salt. These additives, known as diuretics, cause frequent urination and can actually lead to dehydration. Commercial sports drinks can be helpful in preventing dehydration, but in excess cause stomach upset. We recommend a glass of water for every glass of soda, coffee, or other beverage consumed.

Judy's physician recommended that she eliminate all diet sodas to alleviate her joint pain. She replaced her diet sodas with water and, just from this one simple change, her joint pain significantly lessened. It has been suggested that an excessive consumption of diet soda (containing aspartame) over time turns into formaldehyde in the body, which may exacerbate pain.

Some people mistake thirst for hunger. When you feel extremely hungry, start quenching that sensation by drinking water. This will rehydrate your body and prevent you from overeating.

Is it possible to drink too much water? Yes! Avoid excessive water intake over a short period of time. Hyponatremia is a condition of low sodium (salt) in the bloodstream. It results from low amounts of dietary sodium or dilution of sodium by extreme consumption of water. Individuals who are active or exercising over long periods of time are most susceptible. Hyponatremia can lead to life-threatening complications, because your body must carefully balance electrolytes and minerals for proper systemic functioning (cardiovascular, neurological, and musculoskeletal). Excessive intake for each individual varies depending on activity levels. If you require large amounts of water, then balance your intake with an electrolyte drink; for example, follow a glass of water with a cup of a commercial sports drink containing sodium, and continue this cycle as long as you are thirsty.

Creating a Healthy Personal Environment

"You should seek an attractive environment for your energized activities," state Jack Canfield and Mark Victor Hansen in their book *Dare to Win*. The world in which you live is a reflection of you. Immerse yourself in an environment that will facilitate happiness, either individually or with others. Feeling comfortable in your own skin and in your surroundings can help you maintain a positive outlook on life. The following are some tips for creating a healthy physical, mental, and emotional environment.

Physical Environment

- Avoid excessive heat/humidity or cold—play outside on a nice sunny day.

- Limit your exposure to smog, pollution, and cigarette smoke—visit the mountain air.

- While running, avoid hard surfaces (concrete, pavement)—run on a trail in the woods.

- Avoid excess or overindulgence—enjoy exercise, and everything else you do, in moderation.

The Power of Positive Thinking: Veronica's Story (in Her Own Words)

After serving in the U.S. Army for four years, I stopped smoking when I was honorably discharged. Unfortunately, a few months went by, a few pounds were gained, and I was sure it was the result of not smoking. I foolishly started back puffing again.

Years went by and, at twenty-nine, I was smoking one and a half packs per day. I was working in the file room of an x-ray department at a large hospital. It was the evening shift and, when work settled down, the employees that smoked did so in the main control room. At times, there could be four to seven people puffing away, and the room and halls filled with the odor of cigarette smoke.

In July 1984, one of the x-ray technicians who was a nonsmoker and runner, got disgusted enough to approach us. After he lectured us on our terrible habit, he stated that there was a one-mile run the following night. It was a July 4th Celebration Run, which would start at midnight and run out a causeway and back. He didn't think any of us could run one mile and egged us on as we sat there smoking. I thought about the run and how I had wanted to stop my ten-year habit of smoking. Was now the time?

The next night, I hopped in my car, lit up a cigarette, and drove to the race start. I truly believed that running one mile would be no big deal. The gun went off and everybody started running. Well, the race turned out to be a 10K (6.2 miles) and a 3K (1.8 miles). No, not one mile but 1.8 miles, and that 0.8 just about killed me. Coming back off the causeway, the humidity was 100 percent, the temperature was in the eighties, and I had heat problems: I saw sparks going off in my head. I had people twice my age blazing by me like I was standing still. I knew then that if I didn't get my act together about my health, the years ahead were going to be physically difficult. What an eye-opener that night was!

My mind was made up—I stopped smoking that week. It was extremely difficult. I started walking and jogging a few times a week. I went to the YMCA and asked the swimming instructor if I could join the Master's swim group. He said, "If you can swim twenty-five yards, then you can." I swam twenty-five yards and grabbed the wall, wheezing and gasping for air. That week, I started swimming. I eventually worked up to three times a week for seventy-five minutes each class. I was slow, feeling like a gorilla was on my chest, and I was out of shape. But I stuck it out—I didn't want to fail this time.

Three months later, I borrowed a bike and entered my first mini-triathlon. I made it through the eight-mile bike ride, jogged three miles on a beach, and barely survived the eight-mile swim. What a feeling! I was hooked and wanted more.

Nineteen years later, at forty-eight years of age, I can't believe how fortunate I was to be dared to run a "one mile" race. It turned my life around. Over the years, I've competed in more triathlons than I can count, four Ironman races, biathlons, six marathons, swim meets, and distance bike rides. I have logged over 90,000 miles on my bicycle and am in training for ultra-endurance cycling events.

I have had back problems during my athletic endeavors and I was diagnosed with asthma, but at least now I'm exercising, stretching, and doing something about it, instead of sitting on my butt and whining. My point is that if you really want something enough (quitting smoking, losing weight, improving your health) and you believe that it is achievable, you will accomplish your goals. It's all in the mind—believe in yourself, because positive thoughts bring positive results.

Mental Environment

- Avoid negative people and surround yourself with positive people—always smile and offer encouragement.

- Try to limit negative thoughts—think positively.

- Avoid unhealthy behaviors or bad habits.

- Don't be too judgmental of others—treat others as you would like to be treated.

Emotional Environment

- Don't hold a grudge—try to forgive, be patient.

- Avoid anger, hate, and fear—bring more love into your life.

- Avoid isolation for extended periods of time—get out and socialize.

Laughing, Smiling, and Hugging

The average child laughs eighty to a hundred times a day. Can you guess how many times the average adult laughs? The average adult laughs five to seven times per day. What is wrong with this picture? Laughter is currently being researched in several areas of pain management and cancer treatment, focusing on how it may reduce blood pressure and promote relaxation. Some healthcare professionals use laughter and humor in the treatment of injuries and illnesses.

Of course, the state of your health is a serious subject, but don't forget to laugh and smile as much as possible. A lighter heart will enable a stronger mind, body, and soul. Try smiling—not only is it contagious, but it's free. You use thirteen muscles when smiling compared to twenty-eight when frowning. Smiling can improve your quality of life and help to lighten your attitude. Smiling always makes you feel better, and it may make a big difference in the life of someone else, too.

"I love to smile," says Kim. "I always feel good and it brightens the day of everyone I meet—99 percent of the time I get a returned smile. I noticed this effect one day at the gym. I was in the locker room to drop off my bag and, as usual, I smiled at a woman at a nearby locker. She gave me a half-smile and dropped her head. 'Okay,' I thought, 'she's having a bad day.' About an hour later, I reentered the locker room to shower and the same woman was just finishing up with her hair. She came over to me and said, 'I was having a very bad morning—things just weren't going right until you made an incredible effort to reach out with a huge smile. My day turned around for the better and went from bad to good, thank you.' I felt energized the rest of the day."

Not only are we smile deprived, but we are also hug deprived. Hugging is an incredible transfer of energy, offering comfort, security, love, friendship, consolation, and kindness. Most of us want more hugs than we receive, but we're unsure of how to ask for them. We suggest that you hug four people a day to be normal, eight hugs a day for maintenance, and twelve hugs a day for growth. And I mean hug—use your whole body and feel their energy.

"I stopped by the office of my friend and chiropractor one morning to be examined," says Kim. "He would often let me slip in when the patient load was slow. That morning, he had a lobby full of people waiting. I decided at that point to just say 'hi,' grab a quick hug, and leave, but he suggested that I stick around and he would examine me in about thirty minutes. Then, I realized there was someone in the lobby I knew, so I ran over and we hugged and exchanged a few words. At that moment, I noticed that everyone was watching. This was my clue to hug everyone in the lobby—that was what they were waiting for. I smiled and offered hugs to everyone in the lobby. I felt so energized that my back pain disappeared."

Everyone has two choices. We're either full of love or full of fear.
—ALBERT EINSTEIN

Good Sleep Habits

The average adult requires seven to eight hours of sleep a night, but some people try getting away with only three to four hours. How many hours do you get? Sleep is important because it facilitates your body's ability to heal and recover from injury and illness. The body repairs itself during sleep, allowing the immune system to rebuild damaged tissues. Sleep is also your time for cooling down emotionally.

With sleep, the key is consistency. It's important to get the same amount of sleep every night—go to bed around the same time and wake up every morning at the same time. Your body works best on a routine. Sleeping properly and restfully can help prevent disease and illness, so make getting enough sleep a priority and let your body rest and heal itself.

Try not to exercise right before bed, as this can speed up the body's metabolism and keep you from resting properly. End your day by reading a book, saying daily devotions (if appropriate for you), reflecting on the day and yourself. How could you have made it a better day? Go to bed already thinking and believing that tomorrow is going to be better: you will feel good, help people, and do the best job that you can. Say affirmations: be thankful for what this day has brought to you and your loved ones. Deep breathing is helpful for clearing the mind just before dozing off.

Meditation and Visualization

Meditation and visualization are additional tools for strengthening your mind. They can transform your thinking on a daily basis. Meditation can help restore the body to a state of balance. When our bodies experience pain, illness, or injury, we become imbalanced. However, our bodies work constantly to achieve that state of balance (homeostasis) again.

To begin meditating, find a quiet place and begin deep, rhythmic breathing, visualizing some thing or some place that is peaceful and tranquil. When exhaling your breath, focus on relaxing your toes. As soon as your toes are relaxed, concentrate on relaxing your calves (lower leg muscles). Then, move up your body, breathing and relaxing each part, until you reach your neck, shoulders, and head. As you progress, you may want to add affirmations or other positive visualizations.

The key elements of meditation are:

• Posture—either sitting up straight or lying down.

- Breathing—in the belly-breathing technique used during meditation, your breath should distend your lower abdomen, not your chest. Place your hand over your belly button. During the inhalation phase, your hand should rise above your chest—this is proper belly breathing.

- Concentration—thinking, imagining, remembering, fantasizing, processing sensations (touch, smell, sound, sight, taste), visualizing.

It is not uncommon for elite Olympic athletes to spend a great deal of time visualizing their athletic performances months and sometimes years in advance of the competition. They see the end result in their minds, process all of their sensations, and create their own reality. Carl Lewis, Olympic track-and-field competitor, visualized that he would match Jesse Owens's record in the Olympics—and then he did!

We can assist ourselves through visualization exercises, simple tasks that require a small amount of time and can be utilized anytime and anywhere. These exercises can strengthen your focus, reduce tension, stress, and anxiety levels, lower cholesterol and blood pressure, and help battle chronic illness. Perhaps some of you have visualized to some extent already—imagining yourself buying a new car or a bigger house, fantasizing about getting a new job, or seeing a new thinner you in anticipation of losing weight. Use breathing techniques and focus your mind on what is really important in your life and your future; visualizing can be the first step to making it a reality.

"Several years ago, I chaired a committee dedicated to earning national accreditation for my college's athletic-training/sports-medicine education program," recalls Angela. "As the program was developing, I pictured in my mind's eye the dean of our college making congratulatory remarks about our accomplishment at a formal dinner. My vision was so detailed that I could even see the champagne bubbling while the dean was toasting our program's success. As I worked many late nights and weekends, I held on to that vision of achievement. This vision finally became reality just as I had pictured it, including the bubbling champagne!"

THE BALANCING ACT: INCORPORATING COMPONENTS INTO EVERYDAY LIFE (THE FINISHED PRODUCT)

Just like the bumper sticker that reads LIFE IS NOT A DRESS REHEARSAL—LIVE, you must take care of yourself to improve the quality of your life. Your doctor, spouse, family member, or friend is not ultimately responsible for your health—you are! Make yourself a priority in life: schedule time to be with yourself, to pamper and take care of yourself. This does not have to be expensive. Pampering may include weekly or monthly massage, stretching, meditation, facials, or anything that makes you feel good (within legal limits). Take a few minutes before you get out of bed in the morning to stretch, and repeat the stretches before you go to bed. Keep the radio turned off in your car while driving to work and have some quiet time to reflect. Take a personal holiday: one day a month, work half a day and take yourself "out"—go to a movie, go shopping, or just take a drive to your favorite place. Use this time to focus on how your body feels and how you can make yourself feel better, physically, mentally, and emotionally.

Take pride in yourself. If you cannot make yourself happy and healthy, how can you influence others? Have you ever been around someone who is happy and radiates with energy? After talking with that person, you probably felt invigorated. Use this radiant energy from someone else and discover new ways to make changes in your life. Inspire yourself so you can inspire someone else. Continue to strive to make improvements in your outlook, in life, and, most important, in yourself.

Here are some other suggestions for moving toward a healthier lifestyle:

- Stop watching junk TV and switch to educational and inspiring television. Feeding junk TV to yourself can be more hazardous than junk food.

- Take responsibility in all aspects of your life, including finances, health, work, and fun. Remember, balance is the key—when the body is balanced, it's at its peak. Your body sleeps better, heals better, and shines brighter.

- Take more time to read. Reading is educational, inspiring, and motivating. Reading can be done alone or shared with family and friends. Perhaps even join a book club, or create your own. In addition, listening to motivational tapes is easy, cheap, and exhilarating.

- Find a role model, someone you look up to and admire. When people have reached success in life, they typically are excited about sharing with others their stories, experiences, and strategies for success.

- Always remember that you deserve to be relaxed and rested and have time for yourself. If you are having a bad day, lighten it with a present to yourself, such as a massage-therapy appointment.

Are your priorities straight? Our goal is to try to help you seek a balance in your life—body, mind, and soul. Make a list of your priorities and rank them according to importance in your life. Then you can begin to identify where you stand and what imbalances exist in your life. Everyone will have different priorities, but we have listed a few samples below to help get you started:

- Job
- Family
- Spiritual well-being
- Health (mental, physical, emotional)
- Material things (car, house, money, clothes)
- Nonmaterial things (kind acts, charity, tithing)
- Fun activities
- Friends/relationships
- Love

THE MOUNTAIN OF GREATER HEALTH

We have taken you step by step through the process of building a healthier lifestyle to help alleviate your pain. Are you willing to take these steps and prepare for the journey up the mountain of greater health? Use the tools of positive thinking to help you up the mountain: believing in yourself; setting goals and repeating affirmations; healthy habits such as diet, exercise, a healthy environment, humor, sleeping well, meditating and visualizing, and harmonizing your priorities. Throughout this journey, it is our goal to assist you in reaching the summit, leaving you with a healthier body and a more balanced outlook on life. It is now time to *take action*!

BASE CAMP 1 (BC1)

Recognize the signs and symptoms of your pain. Identify and classify the type(s) of pain that you are experiencing. What is the source, or stressor in your life, that's causing your pain? This is the first step for the journey ahead.

BASE CAMP 2 (BC2)

Now that you have recognized your pain, it is time to prepare your mind for its biggest challenge: to believe that your attitude toward pain can be positive. Ground yourself for as long as it takes, protected from the elements, until you believe in yourself and set some positive goals. We have quite a journey ahead and a good attitude will be needed for the higher altitudes.

BASE CAMP 3 (BC3)

Pay attention to your nutritional habits—you'll need sound nutrition and plenty of water to make it up the mountain. Sleep is also very important to help prepare you for the next climb. The mountain can get very tough at this point. With all of these changes occurring, it's a great time to start meditating and visualizing your next step. We will help you incorporate our techniques to facilitate your ascent to the next base camp.

Base Camp 4 (BC4)

What a jump! Through these tough conditions, you have visualized your journey and made it. The next step is to prioritize your time and the important areas of your life. It's like making sure you have all the right gear to make it through the steep climb ahead.

Base Camp 5 (BC5)

You have identified pain, made a leap toward a better attitude, changed to new healthy habits, and begun to relax. Assembling a healthcare team is a valuable tool for reaching true health. Your healthcare team may include a general physician and specialty physician, massage or physical therapist, chiropractor, sports medicine specialist, nutritionist/dietician, strength-and-conditioning specialist/personal trainer, and spiritual counselor (minister, rabbi, priest, psychotherapist). When selecting your healthcare team members, be very choosy: check credentials, licenses, and expertise. We also recommended checking references and speaking to others who have been treated by these professionals. Any member of your healthcare team should support innovative ideas for you and help keep your atmosphere a positive one. We recommend assembling your team ahead of time in order to be prepared. Now, get ready, get set, and go—we are ready for the summit!

Base Camp 6 (BC6)

Congratulations, you have made it! Balancing your act means that you will implement these tools daily, using moderation. Incorporate a little bit at a time, if necessary. Each person is different and will have a singular approach to change.

We simply recommend taking your time and having fun along the way, making it a positive experience. Overindulgence in any aspect of your life may throw you out of balance. If an imbalance occurs, your ability to get better may be hindered or your outlook negatively altered.

Beyond the summit, we will take you on a head-to-toe journey of self-help for your pain. In the following chapters, we will describe in detail the action steps of stretching, strengthening, massage therapy, and other treatments for pain relief.

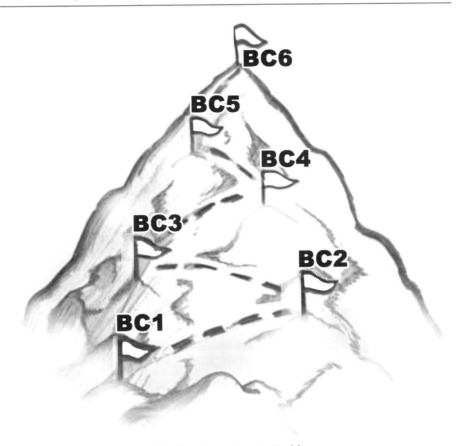

The Mountain of Greater Health

Chapter 3

Take Action Now: The Recipe for Relief

There are a number of therapeutic approaches that have proven highly effective for alleviating pain, including stretching, strengthening exercises, and massage therapy. These can be done with professional guidance or used as self-help techniques for do-it-yourself relief from discomfort. We also describe tips for immediate relief that you can apply to help ease the pain and swelling related to your injury or illness—rest, ice, compression, heat, elevation, and support (aka RICHES). These elements are common therapeutic practices used by most healthcare professionals. In this chapter, we outline the general principles behind these approaches. Chapters 4–9 will then cover specific stretches, exercises, and massage techniques for each area of the body. As you read, remember the importance of becoming proactive: a good understanding of these action steps will help you feel better.

STRETCHING

Muscles attach to bones, and all the bones in the body make up our skeletal system. Within this complex musculoskeletal system are joints, which are made to flex and extend (bend and straighten), and allow for rotation. Our anatomy is what enables us to move in certain directions. The stretching of our muscles allows for our joints to become more flexible. Over a period of time, due to gravity, age (inactivity, tightness, injury, disease), and poor posture, muscles and tendons begin to tighten and shorten, thus limiting our range of motion and decreasing our flexibility. This is comparable to a rubber band that has been weathered for several months—after a while, the rubber band will break when you try to stretch it. Just like the rubber band, your tightened muscles may cause you to walk stiffly with shortened strides, to hunch over when you are seated or standing, or to experience pain as you bend over to tie your shoes.

It's important to note that muscular imbalance contributes to lack of flexibility. For example, affecting the knee joint are the muscles in the front thigh (quadriceps) and the muscles in the back thigh, the hamstring muscles. It is very common to find that the quadriceps are stronger than the hamstrings, due to stress, gravity, spinal conditions, and so on. As a result, you could easily injure the hamstring muscles during activity because of this imbalance.

Stretching daily can relieve tight and tired muscles, bringing new life and elasticity to your soft tissues. Among its other benefits, stretching decreases muscle soreness (especially as we age), encourages exercise, maintains a complete range of motion in our joints (helping prevent injury or stress), and acts as a catalyst to balance the body during the rehabilitation process. As your posture and flexibility improve, your pain levels should decrease, allowing you to feel better all over. Stretching can help you begin to create muscle balance throughout your body. It is beneficial for muscle recovery after exercise and the release of muscle tension and spasm. Studies show that runners who spend time stretching after their workouts show improved muscle recovery compared to those who do not stretch.

Types of Stretching

- *Passive stretching:* This is the type of stretching you're probably most familiar with, which involves holding each stretch for twenty to thirty seconds. This method may cause discomfort and leave you feeling sore.

- *Active Isolated Stretching* (*AIS, or the Mattes Method*): This method follows a unique philosophy regarding stretching. In each stretch, you tighten the opposing muscle (agonist), that is, the muscle opposing the one you are stretching (antagonist). For example, while stretching the back of your upper leg (hamstrings), you actively tighten the front of the leg (quadriceps). You slowly lift the leg, using a rope for an assist, hold for two seconds, and then lower the leg back to the starting position and repeat the exercise (eight to ten repetitions). In this book, we will use AIS as our primary stretching method, because it has proven to be the most effective and least invasive movement technique. Plus, AIS can be accomplished without assistance.

- *Proprioceptive neuromuscular facilitation* (*PNF*): The *agonist-contract method* requires assistance from a partner or therapist. The partner lifts the leg, then the person tightens the leg while the partner applies resistance or a gentle force for five to six seconds. The *hold-relax method* uses the same sequence as above, but following the force applied by the partner, the person will then relax the leg while the partner stretches the muscle to the limit of range of motion. While effective, PNF can often leave the muscle feeling fatigued.

- *Yoga:* This is a meditative exercise that combines flexibility, balance, and relaxation. Yoga is a wonderful way of integrating the mind and body in an activity (mind-body experience). We highly recommend yoga as a way to increase flexibility and access the mind-body experience.

Basic Principles of Active Isolated Stretching

- Never overstretch or stretch violently. Do not take the movement beyond its resistance.

- Never hold a stretch for more than two seconds and always take your stretch back to the starting position.

- Do each stretch eight to ten times.

- Always breathe or exhale your breath when stretching the muscle.

Specific Stretching for Everyone by Aaron Mattes is a great resource for anyone wanting to learn more about proper stretching techniques for injury prevention, rehabilitation, and performance enhancement. Information can also be found on the Internet at the website www.stretchingusa.com. Active Isolated Stretching, the Mattes Method, will be illustrated throughout Chapters 4–9. The instructions and illustrations provide all you need to know to learn self-help techniques encompassing all areas of pain, from nose to toes.

STRENGTHENING EXERCISES: BUILDING ENDURANCE AND POWER

In order to maintain a healthy lifestyle, it is essential to establish or increase total body muscular strength. With muscular strength, you will be more likely to recover from injury and less likely to suffer with soreness. Do you have to be able to lift a Buick to be strong? No. Use your daily activities as a guide for muscle strengthening. Ask yourself the following questions: Can I make it through the day without feeling exhausted? Can I perform regular physical tasks without feeling sore? If I cannot do some activity, is it because of muscular weakness? The good news is that we can all increase our muscular strength regardless of injury, illness, or overall condition.

Numerous studies in exercise physiology have shown that muscle strengthening leads to improvements in other areas, including muscular endurance and muscular power. For most people, muscular endurance is more important because it is needed for carrying out the regular activities of everyday life. And without muscular power, individuals may be limited in their ability to complete daily tasks that require additional strength.

Without muscular strength, endurance, and power, your physical well-being and the quality of your life could diminish. Your posture can be compromised, pos-

Alice's Story

Maintaining physical fitness is not simply a weekend activity but a lifelong endeavor that often calls for adjustments in approach. For years, Alice trained to improve her strength and endurance through competitive rowing, ergometer workouts (exercise equipment that simulates rowing), and running. Unfortunately, this produced stiffness and joint deterioration. More recently, she turned to the study of t'ai chi and yoga to promote flexibility and muscle tone. Despite the benefits of these disciplines, Alice has been slow to overcome nagging persistent "injuries" such as tendinitis, tight hamstrings, heel spurs, and shin splints. "Kim helped me evaluate these issues and prescribed a targeted, easily mastered plan of Active Isolated Stretching that produced results in a few short weeks," says Alice. "AIS is now an essential part of my daily routine."

sibly affecting daily activities such as walking, grocery shopping, proper breathing, and climbing stairs. In other words, your muscles provide a foundation for all bodily movement, including balance and agility.

Increasing your strength, endurance, and power does not require an expensive membership at a fancy health club. Focus on daily activities and use those to strengthen your body (make sure all activities are pre-approved by your healthcare professional):

• Yard work—Do it the old-fashioned way with no riding mower.

• At work—Carry lightweight objects throughout the office; take the stairs instead of the elevator.

• Shopping—Carry your own groceries; park a little farther away.

• Driving—Leave the car at home and use your bicycle or walk.

• Housework—Vacuum, mop, sweep, wash the windows.

Walking the dog around the block is another exercise that can increase your strength, endurance, and power. In Chapter 2, we challenged you to implement a program of 10,000 steps a day. All that is required is an inexpensive pedometer (which measures your steps) and positive motivation. This 10,000-steps challenge is a great way for increasing strength and endurance without spending endless hours at the gym.

In weight lifting, we tend to work the "show muscles" and not the "go muscles." For example, in bodybuilding competitions, weight lifters display what we would consider the "show" muscles—the bigger muscle groups such as leg muscles (hamstrings and quadriceps), chest muscles (pectoralis major and deltoids), biceps and triceps, and back muscles (trapezius and posterior deltoids). Below the surface, you have smaller stabilizing muscles that we call the "go muscles." The body relies heavily on these stabilizing muscles at each joint, but they are not usually as defined as the bigger muscle groups. Weight lifting as it is taught in many local gyms and health clubs also concentrates on the big muscle groups and virtually ignores the "go muscles." Our program will help you condition these stabilizing muscles, which are important in building core strength, helping to prevent injury, and recovering from injury.

In Chapters 4–9, we will provide specific examples of strengthening exercises for each body part. Remember that a key component to muscle strengthening, endurance, and power is balance: when developing your strength routine, remember to work on both sides of your body—right/left and front/back. If you are not sure how to do this, consult a certified strength-and-conditioning specialist (CSCS) for more information.

MASSAGE THERAPY

You probably experienced the simplest form of massage therapy as a child when your mom rubbed the area of your body that you recently hurt, soothing the pain away. Massage therapy is defined as the manipulation of the body's soft tissues, including muscles, tendons, and ligaments. Your mom didn't exactly know what soft tissue she was rubbing, but the pain response was the same: the direct touch not only relaxed the muscle, but also stimulated the release of chemicals in the body known as endorphins, your body's natural painkillers.

What can massage do for you? Aside from making you feel good, massage therapy relieves muscle spasms, increases blood and lymphatic circulation, stimulates immune system function, promotes the healing of soft tissues, increases the relaxation response, and, yes, it can improve your looks.

When the body gets injured, the area of pain swells, which indicates inflammation and tissue damage. In the case of severely injured tissues, massage techniques should not be applied directly to the source of the injury. A gentle massage "milking" the area around the injury can help reduce swelling by acting as a "pumping system" for the muscle tissue to promote the flow of fresh oxygenated blood to the area.

During massage, the therapist gently squeezes the muscle, warming the tissue and promoting blood flow. The systemic, physiological effects of massage are believed to cause the blood to circulate toward the heart. As the tissue is stimulated, the old blood and lymphatic fluid leave the injured area, flow through the lymphatic filtration system, and move toward the heart. As a result of tissue stimulation, the heart sends oxygenated blood to the injury site, thus promoting soft-tissue healing and recovery.

Today, massage therapy is becoming more mainstream in the healthcare industry. In the United States, it is estimated that 28 million people have received a professional massage. Research has shown that as few as two thirty-minute massage sessions per week can significantly reduce pain levels for sufferers of fibromyalgia, arthritis, premenstrual syndrome (PMS), multiple sclerosis, and migraine headaches. In Chapters 4–9, we will introduce specific massage techniques to help assist you in your pain recovery.

When searching for a therapist, be sure to check his or her credentials. About half of the states in the U.S. require licenses; contact the board or department in your area that handles the licensing of massage therapists. Also, seek recommendations from your local massage school and don't be afraid to ask your therapist if he or she is licensed or certified in their field. If you are unsure about their answer regarding licensure or certification, then reconsider using their services.

RICHES

Regardless of whether your pain is acute or chronic, there are general treatment principles that you can apply to help ease the pain and swelling related to an injury or illness. These therapeutic approaches are commonly referred to as RICHES—rest, ice, compression, heat, elevation, and support. Keep in mind that these are general principles and do not replace the advice and expertise of your healthcare professional. Severe sprains or other injuries should always be evaluated by a physician.

Rest

Rest is a period of time of restricted movement or no movement at all, which allows your body to repair the injured tissues. Rest should be monitored according to the initial levels of pain. It would be a great idea to use your pain scale and pain worksheet to monitor your progress (see Figure 1.2 in Chapter 1). Once you feel improvement, you can slowly resume activity. Most minor injuries heal in one to two weeks. For severe injures, consult with your physician first.

Ice

It is almost impossible to go wrong by treating your injury with ice. Cold is particularly recommended for injuries to your musculoskeletal system. A typical treatment lasts approximately twenty minutes. Repeat ice treatments as often as you like, but allow forty minutes of rest between applications. However, prolonged use of ice treatments may cause damage.

Compression

Physically compressing an injured area will help prevent swelling. A common form of compression is an Ace wrap applied around the injured area. Make sure it is not too tight—remember, wraps are not tourniquets. Only apply compression with approval from a healthcare professional.

Heat

Heat may be used for an injury or illness and can be beneficial in relieving tightness and spasm. Make sure you do not apply heat right after the injury occurs: wait for at

Breaking the Pain Cycle

Athletes are very emotional and sensitive when it comes to pain or injury. When athletes come to me (Kim) in pain, they are totally absorbed mentally, emotionally, and physically. They are looking for immediate relief and a quick approval to return to activity. In 1999, I was team therapist for the Zimbabwe track-and-field team during the World Championships in Seville, Spain. While warming up at the track on the morning of competition, one of the runners strained his hamstring. As you might imagine, he was distraught. He was unsure if he could compete that evening. Offering words of encouragement, I worked with him that morning, gently massaging the legs to calm the muscles and promote circulation. In the afternoon, we took a slightly aggressive approach with ice accompanied by gentle massage and AIS. For the remainder of the day, he rested with intermissions of gentle stretching and movement.

By that evening, he felt good enough mentally and emotionally to compete, with a much healthier hamstring. He satisfied himself by running a "good" time and with a new sense of confidence. Giving athletes the opportunity to feel better allows them to focus on healing and lessens the focus on the fact that they are hurt. This is true for anyone experiencing pain. During the cycle of discomfort or immobility, we often focus on what is hurting, the throbbing pain that we are experiencing. Massage therapy combined with stretching has been a great catalyst in breaking the pain cycle.

least seventy-two hours and get approval from your healthcare professional. Apply-ing heat too early in the recovery phase may actually make the injury or illness worse. Do not use heat in the following conditions:

- During the acute stage (the injury has just happened)

- If swelling/discoloration or deformity is present

- If there are signs of infection

- If you are prone to blood clots or have high blood pressure

- When you have an injury or illness that could lead to complications

- Against the advice of your physician

Elevation

Elevation of the injured body part above the heart can help decrease swelling. In this position, gravity can assist in moving fluids back toward the heart.

Support

Support and protection of the injured body part is critical. It may be necessary to purchase protective splints or braces for use during your recovery. Consult your healthcare provider for specific instructions.

You may combine the action steps presented throughout this chapter to facil-itate your recovery, as they often work better as a group. Your healthcare provider should be the final authority regarding your treatment plan.

Remember, don't follow the slogan
"No Pain, No Gain" when you exercise,
lift weights, or play sports.

Always pay attention to your body
and its pain signals.

Chapter 4

Neck and Shoulder Pain

arian is a very active sixty-two-year-old woman who walks three miles every day, travels a great deal, eats carefully to stay slim, and strives to stay "young" and fit. But chronic neck and back pain have bothered her for over five years. She tried massage therapy but the relief was short-lived and, before long, she was in distress again. We taught Marian a series of stretching and flexibility exercises that she can do herself, whether she's at home or traveling, and her life has changed for the better. "I bring diagrams of the relevant stretches wherever I go and practice them daily," she says. "Occasionally I have a massage and flexibility session to 'tune up,' but I arrive at these sessions relaxed instead of in agony. What a nice change!"

NECK PAIN

Neck pain may be caused by tension, stress, or trauma of the cervical spine and the muscles that attach to it. Conditions associated with neck pain include:

- Whiplash/stinger: a traumatic injury caused by violent motion in the neck

- Stress/tension headaches: muscle tightness, trigger points, and weakness in cervical and upper back muscles

- "Crick in the neck": sharp pain on one side, with loss of motion; can be either referred or radiating pain

- Poor posture: muscular weakness, lack of movement, tight chest muscles with rounded shoulders

Sports that subject the athlete's neck to an excessive or violent range of motion, including football, soccer (from heading a ball), rugby, and wrestling, may lead to pain in the cervical spinal region (neck). Car accidents and poor posture (especially

Fun Fact

The human head weighs an average of seven to twelve pounds, depending of the individual. No wonder neck and shoulder muscles get tired and weak—they have to support a lot of weight!

while sitting at a desk, drawing, working on a computer, or talking on the phone) can also contribute to neck pain. In older people, neck pain may be a result of spinal anomalies, arthritis, illness, or spinal disk degeneration. In younger people, neck pain is usually attributed to some type of traumatic injury. Neck pain may also be a symptom of certain illnesses, such as migraine headaches, some types of cancers, lymph/glandular disorders, and circulatory problems. There were over 200,000 cases of neck injuries treated at hospitals throughout the United States in 2001.

Stretching, exercises to strengthen the neck muscles, and massage can all help alleviate neck pain.

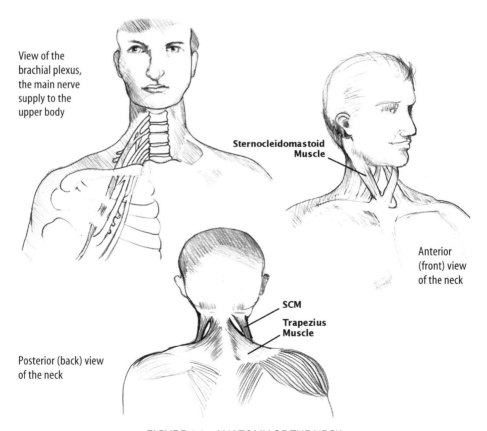

View of the brachial plexus, the main nerve supply to the upper body

Sternocleidomastoid Muscle

Anterior (front) view of the neck

SCM

Trapezius Muscle

Posterior (back) view of the neck

FIGURE 4.1. ANATOMY OF THE NECK

NECK PAIN OVERVIEW	
Signs and Symptoms	**Causes**
• Loss of strength or muscular weakness	• Sleeping in an awkward position
• Loss of motion or movement and stiffness	• Uncomfortable pillows or mattress
• Point tenderness to the touch	• Athletic injury or car accident
• Sharp pain or referred pain	• Poor posture
	• Muscular spasms

Recipe for a Healthy Neck

1. Stretch one to two times daily (morning and evening workouts usually work best); do two sets of eight to ten repetitions, holding each stretch for two seconds only, during each workout. Always take your stretch back to a neutral position before the next repetition; exhale your breath on the stretch phase.

2. Follow your stretching routine with strengthening exercises. These can be repeated two to three times weekly, allowing for one day of rest in between.

3. Practice RICHES: rest, ice, compression, heat, elevation, and support (see Chapter 3).

4. Use hot soaks with Epsom salts (in a bathtub or with a wet cloth) to help reduce neck pain or stiffness.

5. Also effective in lessening pain and stiffness are contrast baths: apply moist heat for five to ten minutes (you can also stretch gently after heat is applied). Moist heat can be applied using a commercial Hydrocollator pack, which is heated in hot water, or a dampened washcloth with a heated gel pack. (We strongly discourage using any type of water treatment with an electric heating pad due to the chance of shock.) Ice, applied for fifteen minutes, should follow the heat application. Always end with a cold application. Repeat this sequence two to three times daily, if necessary.

6. Apply massage techniques one to two times daily.

7. When returning to exercise, stretch lightly for a proper warm-up (use moist heat, if needed). Following exercise, apply ice for fifteen minutes, then stretch again.

8. Maintain a proper diet and hydration for recovery (see Chapter 2).

Stretches for the Neck

A number of stretches have proven effective in promoting flexibility and alleviating neck pain.

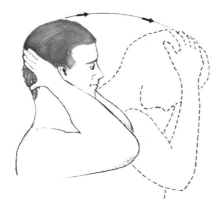

Cervical Flexion

Tuck your chin and move your neck down toward your chest; push gently behind your head for two seconds, exhaling on the stretch phase. Bring your head back to a neutral position. Repeat eight to ten times.

Lateral Flexion (Left Side)

Move your left ear down toward your left shoulder; use your hand to gently assist, and hold for two seconds, exhaling on the stretch phase. Bring your head back to a neutral position. Repeat eight to ten times.

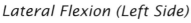

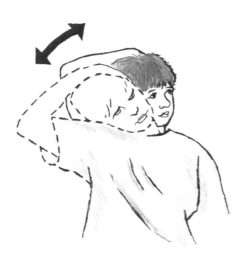

Lateral Flexion (Right Side)

Move your right ear down toward your right shoulder; use your hand to gently assist, and hold for two seconds, exhaling on the stretch phase. Bring your head back to a neutral position. Repeat eight to ten times.

Cervical Hyperextension

Lean forward placing your elbows on your thighs. Extend your head back, gently pushing your chin toward the ceiling (allow your eyes to look up during the stretch phase). Remain leaning forward throughout the movement. Hold for two seconds, exhaling on the stretch phase, and return to the starting position. Repeat eight to ten times.

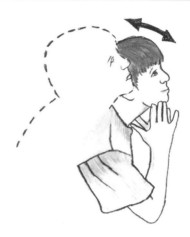

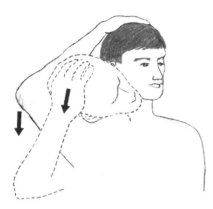

Cervical Oblique Flexion

Turn your head 45 degrees to the right (center your nose over the breast). Move your left ear toward the left side of the breast. Hold for two seconds, exhaling on the stretch phase, and return to the starting position. Repeat eight to ten times. Then, perform the stretch on the other side.

Exercises for the Neck

The following exercises will help you condition your neck muscles and recover from injury.

Head Hyperextension on the Stability Ball

Resting your stomach and chest on the top of the stability ball, start with your head lowered and then slowly raise it. Exhale as you move your head upward. Begin with five repetitions and then gradually increase to fifteen as strength improves.

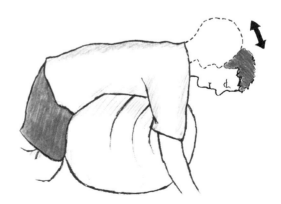

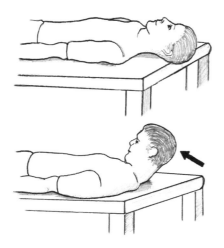

Cervical Flexion

Lying on your back on a table (or the floor), tuck your chin toward your chest and lift your head off the table. Support your head with one hand, if necessary. Exhale on the work phase and repeat ten times.

Note: It is also helpful for the neck to follow the shoulder strengthening routine in the next section.

Massage Technique for the Neck

This massage technique can relieve muscle spasm and pain, increase circulation, and promote the healing of neck injuries.

Assisted Massage for Trapezius, Back of Shoulders, and Neck

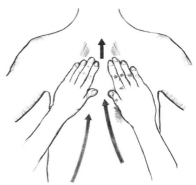

While you are lying on your stomach, the massage assistant glides his or her hands (using the palm surface and fingers) up the trapezius muscle toward the back of the neck, stopping at the base of the skull. Exhale during the gliding phase. Repeat as necessary.

When to Call the Doctor

• If you have persistent pain or swelling

• If you are experiencing shooting pains or numbness

• If you have a continued decrease in your range of motion and strength

Questions and Answers

Q: *Should I use heat or ice?*

A: A good rule of thumb to follow is "When in doubt, always ice!" (unless you have a specific sensitivity to ice). Most health experts would agree that within the first seventy-two hours of an injury, ice is the most effective treatment. Moist heat can be applied after seventy-two hours as long as there is no swelling present in the injured area.

Q: *Can chiropractic adjustments help relieve neck pain?*

A: Absolutely. Chiropractic care can be an important complement to your existing therapy program of stretching, strengthening, and massage. As with selecting any healthcare provider, be sure to check references of a potential chiropractor.

Q: *Should I wear a neck brace?*

A: At the advice or recommendation of your physician, a neck brace may be necessary.

Prevention Is the Key

• Be aware of your posture while sitting, driving, or standing.

• Start out each day with gentle stretching exercises during a warm shower or bath.

• Do strengthening exercises daily.

• Properly warm up before exercise and cool down after exercise.

• Say affirmations: be thankful and appreciative for what each day has brought to you.

SHOULDER PAIN

"A funny thing happened to me on the way into middle age," says Terry. "I could still exercise and do things pretty much the same, but various parts began to ache. No matter how much I tried to ignore these warning signs, they wouldn't go away." Terry had been a runner for years, but heel spurs became too painful for him to continue. He still lifted weights, but he gradually became out of shape, gaining forty pounds. He substituted swimming for running, but soon his shoulders started to ache. Ignoring his pains only meant that his exercise schedule became erratic. "Once I got to the point that I couldn't throw a softball across the room, I knew that I'd better find some relief."

Terry was worried about undergoing shoulder surgery, because friends of his who had the procedure were in more pain afterward. So, he took a chance on massage therapy and his shoulders felt a lot better with regular massages. He also found that massage worked better when he stuck to his regimen of stretching exercises. "I've learned the importance of stretching and flexibility rather than just trying to get stronger," says Terry. "Maybe I am wising up, a little."

Shoulder pain may be caused by overuse, inflammation, stress, or bruising of the muscles surrounding the joint., Conditions associated with shoulder pain include:

- Bursitis: inflammation of the bursa sac in the joint

- Rotator-cuff strain: injury to the muscles or tendons surrounding the joint (The *supraspinatus, infraspinatus,* and *teres minor subscapularis* are the major muscles responsible for the rotator cuff.)

- Trigger points: knots in the muscle, or points of tension and pain, which create a tight or tender spot and often refer pain to another area

- Shoulder tendinitis: inflammation of the tendon in the shoulder, which can cause some "cracking" sounds when the shoulder is moved

- Clicking or grinding: audible sound during movement of the shoulder

Sports or activities, such as baseball, tennis, fly fishing, or swimming, that require repetitive overhead motions may lead to shoulder pain. Even throwing a ball or Frisbee to your dog can cause shoulder injury. Women are typically weaker in the upper

SHOULDER PAIN OVERVIEW

Signs and Symptoms
- Pain when moving the shoulder; tenderness or swelling
- Muscle spasm in the shoulder
- Limitation or loss of range of motion
- Loss of strength or increased weakness
- Cracking or clicking sounds when moving the shoulder joint

Causes
- Overuse injury; excessive overhead motion
- Athletic injury, such as a strain from a throwing or swinging motion
- Poor conditioning or exercising in cold weather with tight muscles
- Bursitis
- Direct trauma or fall

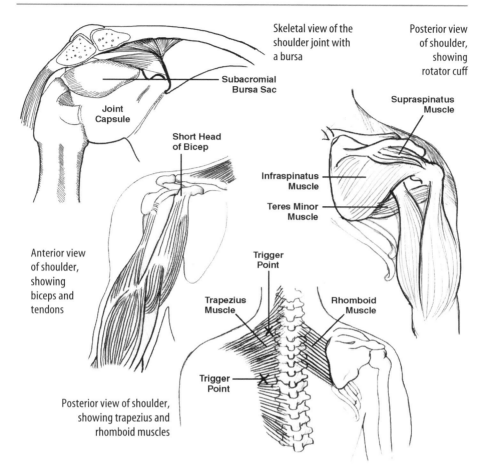

Skeletal view of the shoulder joint with a bursa

Posterior view of shoulder, showing rotator cuff

Subacromial Bursa Sac

Joint Capsule

Short Head of Bicep

Supraspinatus Muscle

Infraspinatus Muscle

Teres Minor Muscle

Anterior view of shoulder, showing biceps and tendons

Trigger Point

Trapezius Muscle

Rhomboid Muscle

Trigger Point

Posterior view of shoulder, showing trapezius and rhomboid muscles

FIGURE 4.2. ANATOMY OF THE SHOULDER

body than men are, and therefore may be more susceptible to shoulder injury. Depending on the activity, women may need more emphasis on strength training to build up the shoulder muscles. It has also been noted that shoulder joints can sometimes be "loose" within the structure of the joint, making them more susceptible to injury with overhead motions or with overuse.

Older individuals may suffer shoulder pain at a higher rate due to conditions such as arthritis, bursitis, and overall atrophy of the shoulder muscle. Also, constantly sleeping on one's side is unhealthy for shoulder joints. Shoulder pain without any specific cause may be a sign of a heart attack.

Stretching, exercises to strengthen the shoulder muscles, and massage can all help alleviate shoulder pain.

Recipe for a Healthy Shoulder

1. Stretch one to two times daily (morning and evening workouts usually work best); do two sets of eight to ten repetitions, holding each stretch for two seconds only, during each workout. Always take your stretch back to the starting position before the next repetition; exhale your breath on the stretch phase.

2. Follow your stretching routine with strengthening exercises. These can be repeated two to three times weekly, allowing for one day of rest in between.

3. Massage with ice two to four times daily for ten minutes each time: Fill a small plastic cup with water and freeze, then peel away the top of the cup so that an inch of the ice is exposed (you can also use a commercially available ice pack, such as Blue Ice). Massage in a circular fashion firmly over the painful shoulder area, always keeping contact with the skin. An ice pack may also be applied to the area without using massage or other movement.

4. Use self-massage techniques to relieve sore muscles.

5. When returning to exercise, stretch gently first (use moist heat, if necessary). If time permits, stretch after exercise, and follow with an ice massage. Gradually increase the amount and intensity of your exercise, as your shoulder will allow.

6. Maintain a proper diet and hydration for recovery (see Chapter 2). Use nutritional supplements, if recommended by your physician.

Stretches for the Shoulder

A number of stretches have proven effective in promoting flexibility and alleviating shoulder pain.

Circumduction

Tighten your stomach, lean forward slightly, and slightly bend your knees. Move your arms in small circles, gradually increasing the size of the circles. Breathe evenly during movements.

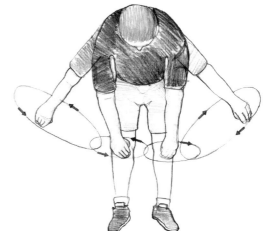

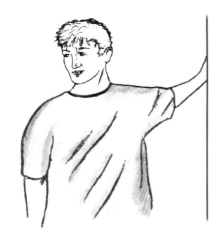

Chest Muscle Stretch

Place the palm of your right hand on a doorframe or wall (any stabilizing surface will do). Gently rotate your torso (upper body/trunk) toward your left side to stretch the chest muscle. Remember to assist yourself through the movement by contracting the back of the shoulder as you rotate your torso. Hold for two seconds, exhaling on the stretch phase, and return to the starting position. Repeat eight to ten times. Then, perform the stretch on the other side.

Biceps Tendon/Anterior Shoulder Stretch

While seated, tuck your chin slightly toward your chest and lean slightly forward. Keep your arms close to your sides. With thumbs pointed down, move your arms straight back. Hold for two seconds, exhaling on the stretch phase, and return to the starting position. Repeat eight to ten times.

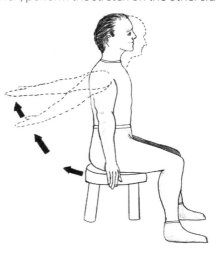

Rotator Cuff (External) Stretch

Keeping your arms level with your shoulders, bend your elbows to 95 degrees. Palms face down at the beginning. Rotate your arm backward (externally) as far as possible. Hold for two seconds, exhaling on the stretch phase, and return to the starting position. Repeat eight to ten times.

Rotator Cuff (Internal) Stretch

Keeping your arms level with your shoulders, bend your elbows to 90 degrees. Palms face down at the beginning. Rotate your arm downward (internally) as far as possible. Hold for two seconds, exhaling on the stretch phase, and return to starting position. Repeat eight to ten times.

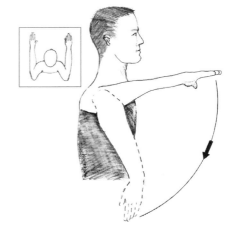

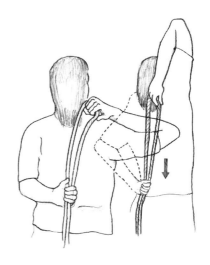

Horizontal Flexion

Standing with your arms at your sides, keep your right elbow straight with your thumb pointed up. Bring your right arm across and toward the top of the left shoulder. Place your left hand at the right elbow and gently use it to assist moving your arm toward the top of the left shoulder. Hold for two seconds, exhaling on the stretch phase, and return to the starting position. Repeat eight to ten times. Then, perform the stretch on your other side, extending the left arm.

Triceps Stretch

At the starting position, flex your left elbow behind your back, keeping your forearm parallel to the floor with the palm facing outward. Holding a length of rope, reach your right arm vertically over the right shoulder. Grab the rope with your left hand and pull down gently to assist the stretch. Hold for two seconds, exhaling on the stretch phase, and return to the starting position. Repeat eight to ten times. Then, perform the stretch on the other side.

Exercises for the Shoulder

The following exercises will help you condition your shoulder muscles and recover from injury.

Anterior Fly

Lie on your back on the floor or on a bench with arms extended out to the sides. Inhale your breath. Then, using lightweight dumbbells, bring

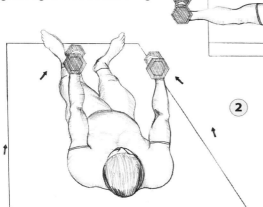

the weights up so that your arms extend straight above your shoulders. Exhale your breath as you lift the weights. Slowly lower the weights to the starting position. Repeat ten times. Add more weight as necessary.

Forward Extension

Begin in a seated position, with arms by your sides and holding light dumbbells (palms facing the body). Raise your arms straight in front of you, keeping your arms in line with the shoulders. Exhale your breath as you lift the weights. Slowly lower the weights to the starting position. Repeat ten times. Add more weight as necessary.

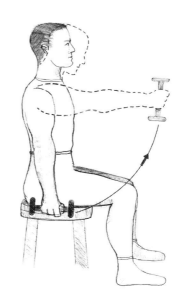

Shoulder Abduction

Begin in a seated position, with arms by your sides and holding light dumbbells (palms facing the body). Lift your arms out from your body to the sides toward shoulder level. Exhale your breath as you lift the weights. Slowly lower the weights to the starting position. Repeat ten times. Add more weight as necessary.

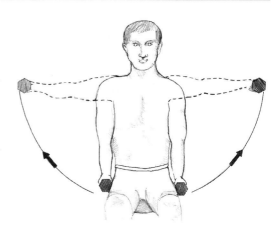

Rotator Cuff (Internal)

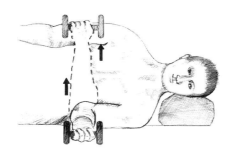

Begin lying on your left side. Holding a light dumbbell in your left hand, bend your left elbow to a 90-degree angle, with forearm parallel to the floor and upper arm held against the body. Lift the weight until it reaches the right side of your body (maintain a 90-degree angle). Exhale your breath as you lift the weight. Slowly lower the weight to the starting position. Repeat ten times. Then do the same exercise on the right side. Add more weight as necessary.

Rotator Cuff (External)

Begin lying on your left side. Bend your top (right) elbow to a 90-degree angle and hold across the body, with a light dumbbell in your hand. Use a small cushion or pad under the right elbow. Raise the arm upward slowly (maintaining a 90-degree angle). Exhale your breath as you lift the weight. Slowly lower the weight to the starting position. Repeat ten times. Then do the same exercise on the other side. Add more weight as necessary.

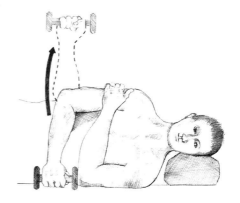

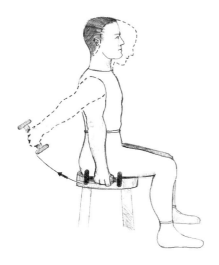

Posterior Extension

Begin seated with arms by your sides, palms facing the body and holding light dumbbells. Tuck chin, lean forward slightly, and lift the arms backwards (elbows straight) as high as possible. Exhale your breath as you lift the weight. Slowly lower your arms to the starting position. Repeat ten times. Add more weight as necessary.

Shoulder Shrugs

Begin with arms at your sides, palms facing the body and holding light dumbbells. Then shrug your shoulders forward, then upward, and finally backward. Exhale your breath on the work phase. Slowly lower your arms to the starting position. Repeat ten times. Add more weight as necessary.

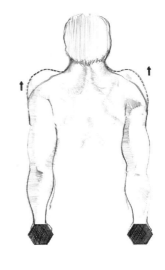

Triceps Extension

Lie face-up on a bench. Grip a dumbbell in each hand and rest them on either side of your head, with your elbows bent above you. Exhale and lift both arms until extended above you. Hold for two seconds and return to the starting position. Repeat fifteen times. Add more weight as necessary.

Massage Techniques for the Shoulders

These massage techniques can relieve muscle spasm and pain, increase circulation, and promote the healing of shoulder injuries.

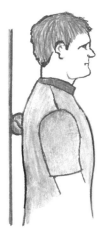

Tennis Ball to Rhomboids Against Wall

This technique helps reduce pain between the shoulder blades. Place a tennis ball between your back and a wall, with the ball located between the spine and the shoulder blade. (Do not place the ball directly on the spine.) Lean back gently and roll the ball up and down a few inches on each side of the spine. This technique will require you to squat slightly with your legs. Try this for a few minutes at a time to help relieve tight muscles and spasms.

Friction to Shoulder (Deltoid Tendon or Biceps Tendon)

Place the tips of your fingers directly on the sore area. Press down firmly into the muscle and make small circular movements or side-to-side motions. Let the level of pain be your guide in how much pressure to use. After a few minutes, stretch and then ice massage. Repeat as necessary.

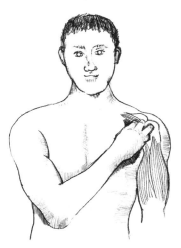

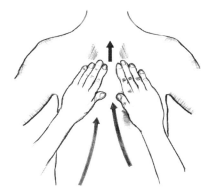

Assisted Massage for Back of Shoulders, Trapezius Muscle, and Neck

While you are lying on your stomach, the massage assistant glides his or her hands (using the palm surface) up the trapezius muscle toward the back of the neck. Exhale during the gliding phase. Repeat as necessary.

When to Call the Doctor

- If you have persistent swelling or pain (localized or radiating)

- If you have lack of movement or decreased range of motion

- If you develop a "frozen" shoulder—when the joint is restricted by scar tissue, muscular pain, and spasm

- If you feel numbness or tingling in the shoulder or down your arm

- If you experience a loss of strength in the shoulder or arm

Questions and Answers

Q: *What causes trigger points (knots) and how do I get rid of them?*

A: Poor posture (shoulders rolled forward), overuse or overexertion of shoulder muscles, and trauma can cause trigger points in the back of the shoulder area or between the shoulder blades. Trigger points can be very painful and sometimes cause referred pain or discomfort.

Here's an analogy of what the muscle tissue does when it's overworked, tired, or stressed: Imagine your muscles as a fresh stack of pancakes, hot off the griddle. The pancakes are typically very fluffy and stacked high. The body is also made in layers of muscles—when muscle tissue is "healthy" or "fresh," it is also fluffy. And just like a stack of pancakes left out on the counter for a day, your muscles flatten out and stick together when they are overworked. At this point, they form little adhesions or "trigger points," otherwise known as knots.

The best way to eliminate trigger points is to stretch daily, maintain proper posture, and exercise daily. This keeps your muscles really fresh and stress-free. Massage therapy or trigger-point therapy are also useful tools if you already have knots. These types of therapy can be self-administered or professionally done (depending on the severity of pain you are experiencing). Acupuncture and chiropractic can also be helpful, along with icing.

Q: *I wake up with shoulder pain and some numbness each morning. Is this normal?*

A: Typically, sleeping on your side restricts proper blood flow and nerve supply to the shoulder joint. There are also tiny stabilizing muscles and muscle attachments that stay contracted when you lie on your side—as a result, they limit the amount of blood and nerve impulses to the rest of the arm. These would be the first considerations, but since there could be other underlying causes, you should seek the attention of a physician.

> **Q:** *Is carrying a heavy briefcase, laptop, or book bag harmful?*
>
> **A:** Yes, carrying luggage, especially on one side of the body, can be very harmful and cause an imbalance of muscle tissues. This is not only harmful to your shoulders, but can be potentially harmful to your low back. Some suggestions for remedying this are:
>
> • Use wheels and roll your luggage on the ground.
>
> • Lighten your load—do you need everything in your bag?
>
> • Share the load—switch sides of the body frequently or get help carrying heavy items.
>
> • Invest in a high-quality backpack.

Prevention Is the Key

• Stretch daily!

• Warm up before participating in sports and properly cool down afterward.

• Increase your body awareness—pay attention to any warning signs throughout your body, including pain, loss of motion, muscular atrophy, or numbness.

• If you are participating in sports, use proper techniques and movements.

• Make sure all sporting equipment fits you correctly.

Chapter 5

Torso Pain

A young client of Kim's suffered an unfortunate surgical outcome three years ago. At the age of fifteen, Lisa underwent back surgery to correct her spinal misalignment, caused by severe scoliosis. On the morning of her surgery she entered the hospital walking. Weeks later, she left the hospital confined to a wheelchair. There were some complications during surgery that resulted in the loss of her lower-body function. It has been a long and difficult road for this young girl over the years, but because of her willingness to remain positive, her abilities have improved immeasurably. She suffers from severe muscle spasms in her trunk/torso/abdominal area and lower legs. These spasms can be very painful and frightening, sometimes causing an inability to move her trunk. We have spent many hours teaching her how to stretch her upper body (torso, trunk, abdominals, neck, and shoulders) while being restricted to her wheelchair. The stretching exercises have helped her control or eliminate the spasms in her torso, thus controlling or eliminating her pain. In addition, she has learned several "wheelchair" strengthening exercises. She now is able to transfer herself to her own bed, therapy table, and bathtub. She has maintained a great attitude, willingness to learn, and tremendous self-esteem. "My confidence has helped me to be strong since the surgery and it has made me look at life in a different way. I am so appreciative of the tools that I have acquired to keep my life comfortable and strong."

Torso or trunk pain may be the result of direct trauma or strain to the chest, ribs, or stomach. This might involve an injury to the soft tissues, such as muscles, tendons, or ligaments. Conditions associated with torso pain include:

• Abdominal or chest strain: sore or injured chest or stomach muscle causing discomfort when lying on the stomach or moving from a seated to a standing position

- "Stitch in side": cramplike pain in the side of the trunk or the ribs—possibly due to trauma or lack of oxygen to the diaphragm (poor breathing technique)

- Sharp abdominal pain on the lower right side: possibly appendix pain or a rupture—see a physician immediately

- Bruised ribs: soreness or pain in the ribcage caused by direct force, falling, or repetitive or explosive movement (such as weight lifting or rowing)

- "Getting the wind knocked out of you": temporary breathing difficulty caused by direct force to the diaphragm or falling down.

Torso pain could indicate respiratory or cardiac problems as well as internal organ injury. According to the National Electronic Injury Surveillance System (NEISS), approximately 500,000 injuries to the upper trunk, involving an emergency-room visit, occurred in the United States in 2001.

Stretching, exercises to strengthen the torso, and massage can all help alleviate torso pain.

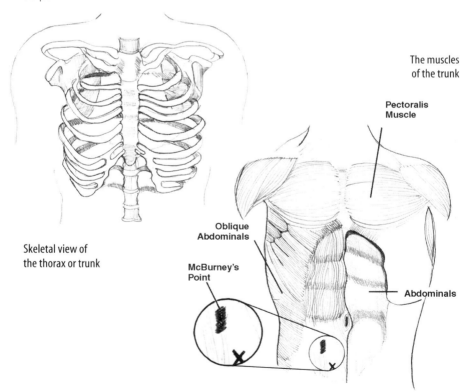

The muscles of the trunk

Pectoralis Muscle

Oblique Abdominals

McBurney's Point

Abdominals

Skeletal view of the thorax or trunk

FIGURE 5.1. ANATOMY OF THE TORSO

TORSO PAIN OVERVIEW

Signs and Symptoms

- Spasm or cramping of the abdominal muscles and side of the body
- Trouble breathing or unusual sounds on inhalation and exhalation
- Dull, sharp, or localized pain (during inhalation or when twisting the torso)
- Blood in urine or coughing up blood (associated with internal injury)
- Discoloration/bruising or deformity of injured area
- Swelling or tenderness
- Pain when sneezing or coughing
- Pain in the abdomen

Causes

- Direct trauma/injury or falling down
- Poor breathing technique
- Internal causes (hemorrhaging, disease, trauma)
- Poor muscle conditioning or strength
- Poor equipment or technique for athletics or weight lifting
- Appendicitis

Recipe for a Healthy Torso

1. Start each morning with postural exercises (standing or seated) using belly breathing; focus on proper breathing techniques.

2. Stretch gently one to two times daily; hold each stretch for two seconds only. Return to the starting position before the next repetition (perform eight to ten repetitions); exhale your breath on the stretch phase.

3. Perform RICHES: rest, ice, compression, heat, elevation, and support (see Chapter 3).

4. Strengthening exercises can be done two to three times weekly, with one day of rest in between. It is important to always stretch before you strengthen.

5. Self-massage techniques can be applied one to two times daily.

6. When returning to exercise, stretch first as part of your warm-up. Practice proper breathing techniques while exercising and gradually increase exercise intensity as symptoms improve. Afterward, cool down with stretches and ice (if necessary). Any pain and discomfort should be an indication to stop exercising immediately.

7. Undergo nutritional recovery. Eat extra fiber to avoid constipation if you've been sedentary, and make sure you achieve proper hydration (see Chapter 2).

8. If you are a smoker, quit.

9. Avoid painful movements. If pain persists, seek physician care promptly.

Stretches for the Torso

A number of stretches have proven effective in promoting flexibility and alleviating torso pain.

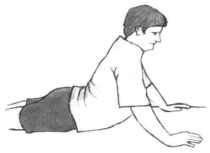

Abdominal Stretch

Lie on your stomach and place your hands (palms down) at your shoulders. Contract your back muscles and gently raise your torso up from the floor, using your arms to assist. Exhale on the stretch phase and hold for two seconds, then return to the starting position. Repeat eight to ten times.

Seated Low-Back Stretch

Sit with your knees shoulder-width apart and toes pointed straight ahead. Tuck your chin in and contract your abdominal muscles, then slowly bend forward toward the floor. Do not bounce at the end of the movement. Exhale on the stretch phase and hold for two seconds, then return to the starting position. Repeat eight to ten times.

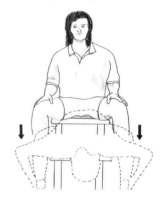

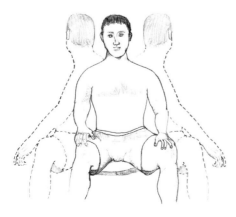

Trunk Rotation

While seated, keep your hips pointed forward and gently rotate your torso to the right. Reach your right hand behind you, while the left hand assists with the rotation by gently pressing against your right leg. Exhale on the stretch phase and hold for two seconds, then return to the starting position. Repeat ten times. Then, perform the same stretch on the left side.

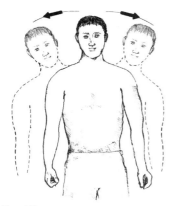

Lateral Flexion of the Torso

Stand with your feet shoulder-width apart. Your hands are relaxed at your sides, with palms facing toward the body. Slowly bend sideways to the left as far as possible. Exhale on the stretch phase and hold for two seconds, then return to the starting position. Repeat eight to ten times. Then, perform the same stretch on the right side.

Hip Flexor

Kneel with your right knee on the floor (place a pad under the knee). Your left leg is bent at the knee with your foot flat on the ground about twelve inches in front of the left knee. Lean forward onto the flexed (left) knee until the knee is directly above your left ankle. Contract your stomach muscles as you do this movement. Exhale on the stretch phase and hold for two sec-

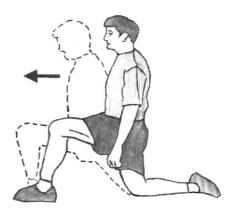

onds, then return to the starting position. Repeat eight to ten times. Then, perform the same stretch with the left knee on the floor and the right knee extended.

Exercises for the Torso

The following exercises will help you condition your torso muscles and recover from injury.

Oblique Abdominal Muscles

Lie on your back with your knees bent and place one hand behind your head. Lift up and move your elbow toward the opposite knee. Return to the starting position and repeat ten times. Then, perform the same exercise on the other side.

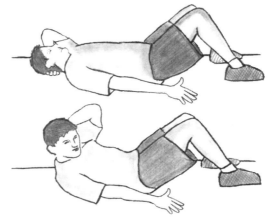

Abdominal Crunches

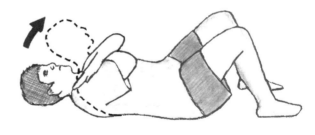

Lie on your back with your knees bent and cross your arms on your chest. Slowly lift your upper body, aiming your chin toward your belly button (keep your chin slightly tucked). Keep your pelvis tilted back toward the floor and exhale as you do the exercise. (If your abdominal muscles are too weak at first, grip under your thighs to assist lifting your upper body.) Return to the starting position and repeat fifteen times.

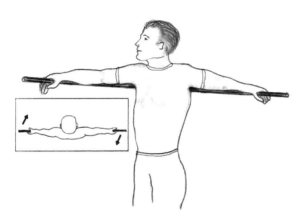

Standing Trunk Rotation with Bar

Holding a bar or broomstick, and standing with your feet shoulder-width apart, rotate slowly in one direction and then the other. Concentrate on using your oblique muscles (sides of the abdomen). Exhale as you move to each side and repeat ten times.

Lateral Flexion with Dumbbells

Stand with both arms by your sides, palms facing the body and one hand holding a light dumbbell. Slowly bend to the side with the weight. Exhale as you return to the starting position. Repeat ten to fifteen times and then exercise the other side. Add more weight as necessary.

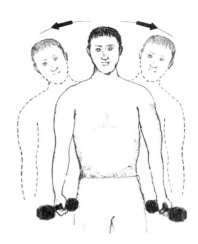

Half Superman

Lie on your stomach on a table or mat. Lift your left arm and right leg simultaneously, then switch to lifting your right arm and left leg. As your strength improves, you can add weights (to wrists and ankles). Start with five repetitions and increase as you get stronger. Movements should be very slow and controlled; exhale on the work phase.

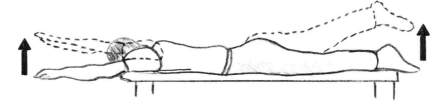

Massage Techniques for the Torso

These massage techniques can relieve muscle spasm and pain, increase circulation, and promote the healing of torso injuries.

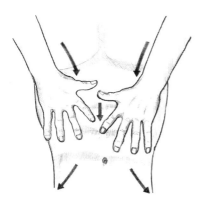

Gliding Abdominal Massage

While lying on your back, glide both your hands downward on the abdominal muscles, using the palm surface, with lotion or massage oil. Start just under the chest and reach for the belly button. Exhale through the movement; repeat as necessary.

Assisted Diaphragmatic Maneuver

While you are lying on your back, the massage assistant gently places his or her thumbs at the bottom of your rib cage. Exhale as the assistant glides his or her thumbs along the diaphragm under the rib cage. Repeat a few times, being sure to exhale your breath deeply during the massage.

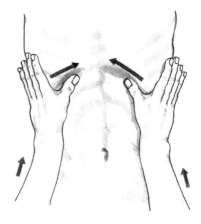

Postural/Breathing Exercises

Proper posture is important to help reeducate and realign your spine. It's important to employ proper breathing while practicing postural exercises. When breathing correctly, your diaphragm muscle (located under the rib cage) is responsible for the proper inhalation and exhalation of your lungs. Shallow breathing employs the chest muscles, thus placing undue stress and/or strain to the muscles located between the shoulders and in the neck. (Shallow breathing can develop into trigger points and chronic neck/shoulder pain.)

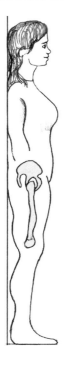

Standing Postural Exercise

Stand against a wall, with your low back (requires a pelvic tilt), shoulders, and back of head touching the wall. Hold the position for a minute, breathing deeply through the exercise, then relax and repeat as necessary. This position will feel awkward at first, but it will help retrain your body for a better posture.

Seated Postural Exercise

While seated, tilt your pelvis slightly backward. Bring your shoulders back and maintain a 90-degree flexion at the hips and knees. (If needed, place a phone book under your feet to achieve the proper angles for hips and knees.) Hold the position for a minute, breathing deeply through the exercise, then relax and repeat as necessary.

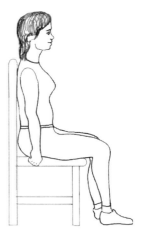

Belly Breathing Exercise

While lying on your back, place your hand on top of your belly button. Take a deep breath, breathing in through your nose and into your belly. Your hand should rise

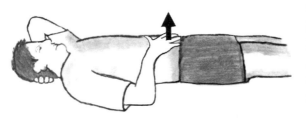

above your chest upon inhalation. Then, exhale your breath through your mouth. As you breathe, concentrate on relaxing your toes first, then your lower legs, your upper legs next, and so on until you reach the top of your head, reducing tension in each part of your body. Not only does this exercise teach you proper breathing, but it can also help initiate relaxation. Try to practice this breathing exercise every day.

When to Call the Doctor

- If you experience chronic coughing or difficulty in breathing

- If there is persistent sharp pain or swelling in the abdomen

- If you have a fever or are vomiting

- If there is blood in your urine or you are coughing up blood

Questions and Answers

Q: *What are some additional activities that could help me strengthen my upper body or torso?*

A: We have found that swimming offers a variety of benefits: it increases the strength and endurance of the whole body, encourages proper breathing techniques, provides a weightless environment for exercise (which is helpful to injured joints), and feels good all over. Other activities for building upper-body strength include t'ai chi and martial arts.

Q: *Last month, I injured my chest muscle at the breast bone while lifting weights in the gym. When can I get back to lifting weights?*

A: Depending on the severity of the strain, allow four to six weeks for recovery. The classifications of strains are:

Mild: slightly pulled muscle; no loss of strength or tearing

Moderate: some slight tearing of the muscle or tendons; significant loss of strength

Severe: complete tear or rupture of the muscle, tendons, or cartilage

For moderate to severe strains, your recovery process may be longer. Please seek advice and direction from your physician if this is the case. Possible bruising may be present. Upon returning to exercise, allow pain to guide you through your activity. A qualified strength-and-conditioning coach or a physical trainer can check for proper form and correct amount of weight. During the recovery phase, gentle stretching and icing are helpful in lessening the recovery time. It's important to following stretching with some gentle strengthening to re-create a core balance of chest muscles.

Q: *What does getting the "wind knocked out of me" mean?*

A: Typically, this injury is known as trauma to the solar plexus (a bundle of nerves around the belly button). As a result of direct trauma, the diaphragm becomes temporarily paralyzed, causing difficulty in breathing. Fear and anxiety can worsen symptoms; therefore, it's important to practice staying calm using proper breathing techniques. If symptoms persist or worsen, seek professional medical attention immediately.

Hyperventilation Relief

Hyperventilation, an excessive rate of inhalation and exhalation, is usually due to anxiety-induced stress or asthma. This leads to an abnormal loss of carbon dioxide from the blood. Signs and symptoms of this condition include wheezing, difficulty in getting air, or gasping for air. The first goal in alleviating hyperventilation is to decrease the rate of carbon dioxide loss. Try to slow down the breathing rate of the person suffering from hyperventilation. This can be accomplished by having the person breathe in through their nose and exhale through their mouth. Another technique is to have the person inhale and exhale through one nostril while pinching the other nostril off and keeping the mouth closed. A third technique is breathing into a paper bag.

Prevention Is the Key

- Good nutrition and adequate hydration is critical.

- Practice proper breathing techniques during activity and at rest.

- Use the right equipment for your sport or activity; get instructions and use proper techniques.

- Be sure to warm up before exercise and cool down afterward.

- Increase your body awareness—pay attention to any warning signs throughout your body, including pain, loss of motion, muscular atrophy, or numbness.

Chapter 6

Pain in the Arm, Wrist, and Hand

As a certified athletic trainer, I (Angela) have treated many athletes with an inflammatory condition of the elbow called epicondylitis: pain on the inside (medial) or outside (lateral) areas of the elbow. This condition is usually caused by overuse. I administer several sports medicine treatments, including icing the area, stretching the arm muscles, applying heat, ultrasound, a tension elbow strap, and referral to a physician for a prescription of anti-inflammatory drugs. The athletes with epicondylitis progress slowly, but being a persistent athletic trainer, I often broaden my therapy regimen to include massage therapy and chiropractic care. This more holistic approach facilitates a speedier recovery for these athletes.

ARM PAIN

Arm pain may be the result of direct trauma or injury (repetitive stress or overuse) to the muscles or ligaments surrounding the elbow, shoulder, and wrist joints. Conditions associated with arm pain include:

- "Tennis elbow" or "golfer's elbow": inflammation of the muscles, tendons, or bursa surrounding the elbow joint (Tennis elbow is pain at the outside of the elbow joint; golfer's elbow is pain at the inside of the elbow joint.)

- Arm bruise: discoloration and bruising of the soft tissue of the upper arm and forearm

- Bicipital tendinitis: inflammation of a biceps tendon in the upper arm in front of shoulder

Activities involving repetitive motion, such as throwing a ball, overhead motions in swimming or volleyball, or handling weighted objects in awkward positions (stocking shelves at a store, for example) are common causes of arm pain. Arm pain may also be a symptom of heart or circulatory problems. It is estimated that there were over 300,000 cases of upper- and lower-arm injuries in the United States in 2001.

Stretching, exercises to strengthen the arm muscles, and massage can all help alleviate arm pain.

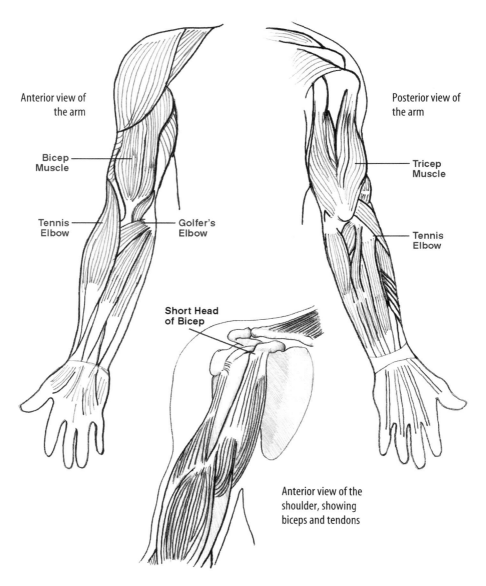

FIGURE 6.1. ANATOMY OF THE ARM

ARM PAIN OVERVIEW

Signs and Symptoms	*Causes*
• Tightness or weakness	• Repetitive stress from activity (either sports-related or work-related)
• Aching elbow or arm	• Strain from overuse
• Radiating pain throughout the elbow and arm	• Micro tear in the tendon of the muscle attached at the joint
• Painful and decreased motion	• Poor techniques while playing sports
• Swelling	• Improper athletic equipment (weight, tension, grip)

Recipe for a Healthy Arm

1. Stretch one to two times daily (especially before and after activity); do eight to ten repetitions, holding each stretch for two seconds only. Always take your stretch back to the starting position before the next repetition; exhale your breath on the stretch phase.

2. Strengthening exercises can be done two to three times per week. Always allow for a rest day in between sessions. Remember to stretch before you strengthen.

3. For acute pain, massage with ice two to four times daily for ten minutes each time: Fill a small plastic cup with water and freeze, then peel away the top of the cup so that an inch of the ice is exposed (you can also use a commercially available ice pack, such as Blue Ice). Massage in a circular fashion firmly over the affected area, always keeping contact with the skin.

4. Rest or limit activities for a period of time, if necessary.

5. Massage therapy, or friction to the tendon area, can be applied one to two times daily; you may consider icing afterward.

6. When returning to exercise or activity, stretch and warm up first. Gradually increase exercise as symptoms or pain lessens. An elbow strap may be necessary to help ease the pressure while exercising. Remember to always cool down and apply ice when finished.

7. Maintain a proper diet and hydration for recovery (see Chapter 2).

8. If inflammation is present, anti-inflammatory medications may be necessary.

Stretches for the Arm

A number of stretches have proven effective in promoting flexibility and alleviating arm pain.

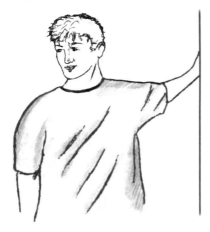

Chest Muscle Stretch

Place the palm of your right hand on a doorframe or wall (any stabilizing surface will do). Gently rotate your torso (upper body/trunk) toward your left side to stretch the chest muscle. Remember to assist yourself through the movement by contracting the back of the shoulder as you rotate your torso. Hold for two seconds, exhaling on the stretch phase, and return to the starting position. Repeat eight to ten times. Then, perform the stretch on the other side.

Biceps Tendon/Anterior Shoulder Stretch

While seated, tuck your chin slightly toward your chest and lean slightly forward. Keep your arms close to your sides. With thumbs pointed down, move your arms straight back. Hold for two seconds, exhaling on the stretch phase, and return to the starting position. Repeat eight to ten times.

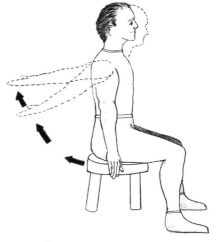

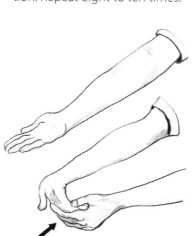

Forearm/Wrist Extension I

Hold your right arm out straight with the palm facing up. Grip the fingers of your right hand with your other hand and gently bend them downward and back. Hold for two seconds, exhaling on the stretch phase, and return to the starting position. Repeat eight to ten times. Then, perform the stretch on the left arm.

Forearm/Wrist Extension II

Hold your left arm out straight with the palm facing down. Extend the fingers up and back, assisting with your other hand to gently bend the palm and fingers of the left hand. Hold for two seconds, exhaling on the stretch phase, and return to the starting position. Repeat eight to ten times. Then, perform the stretch on the right arm.

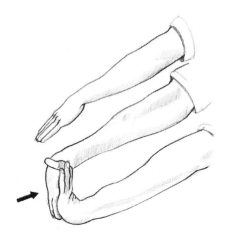

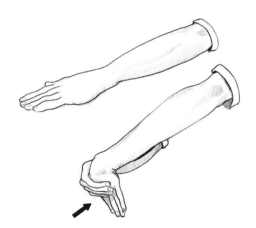

Forearm/Wrist Flexion I

Hold your left arm out straight with the palm facing down. Flex the wrist downward, assisting with your other hand to gently bend the left wrist. Hold for two seconds, exhaling on the stretch phase, and return to the starting position. Repeat eight to ten times. Then, perform the stretch on the right arm.

Forearm/Wrist Flexion II

Hold your left arm out straight and make a fist. Flex the wrist downward, assisting with your other hand to gently bend the left wrist. Hold for two seconds, exhaling on the stretch phase, and return to the starting position. Repeat eight to ten times. Then, perform the stretch on the right arm.

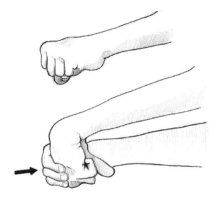

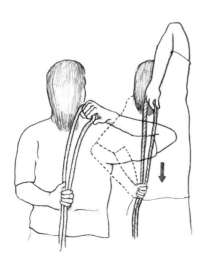

Triceps Stretch

At the starting position, flex your left elbow behind your back, keeping your forearm parallel to the floor with the palm facing outward. Holding a length of rope, reach your right arm vertically over the right shoulder. Grab the rope with your left hand and pull down gently to assist the stretch. Hold for two seconds, exhaling on the stretch phase, and return to the starting position. Repeat eight to ten times. Then, perform the stretch on the other side.

Ulnar Flexion

Hold out your right arm in front of you, keeping the elbow extended and the palm facing down. Use your other hand as shown and flex the wrist gently toward the little-finger side. Hold for two seconds, exhaling on the stretch phase, and return to the starting position. Repeat eight to ten times. Then, perform the stretch on the left arm.

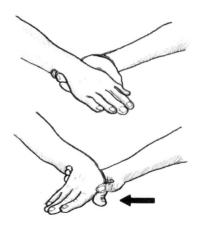

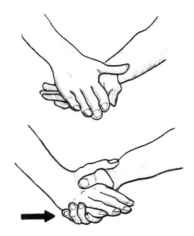

Radial Flexion

Hold out your right arm in front of you, keeping the elbow extended and the palm facing down. Use your other hand as shown and flex the wrist gently toward the thumb side. Hold for two seconds, exhaling on the stretch phase, and return to the starting position. Repeat eight to ten times. Then, perform the stretch on the left arm.

Exercises for the Arm

The following exercises will help you condition your arm muscles and recover from injury.

Wrist Extension

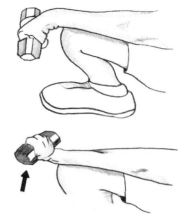

Support your arm on the thigh, palm facing down and holding a light dumbbell. Extend the wrist up and back as far as it will go. Keep your grip as relaxed as possible, and exhale on the work phase. Hold the extension for two seconds and return to the starting position. Repeat fifteen times. Then, perform the lift with the other arm. Add more weight as necessary.

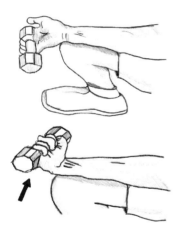
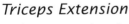

Wrist Flexion

Support your arm on the thigh, palm facing up and holding a light dumbbell. Start with your grip relaxed and hand hanging down over your knee. Flex your wrist toward you as far as it will go, exhaling on the work phase. Hold for two seconds and return to the starting position. Repeat fifteen times. Then, perform the lift with the other arm. Add more weight as necessary.

Triceps Extension

Lie face-up on a bench. Grip a dumbbell in each hand and rest them on either side of your head, with your elbows bent above you. Exhale and lift both arms until extended above you. Hold for two seconds and return to the starting position. Repeat fifteen times. Add more weight as necessary.

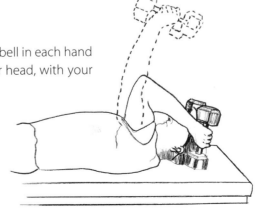

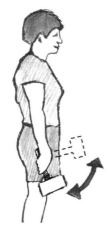

Flexion of Forearm (Front)

Standing, grasp a weighted bar or hammer, with the weighted end in front of you. Flex your wrist by lifting the weight toward the ceiling without moving the arm, exhaling on the work phase. Hold for two seconds and return to the starting position. Repeat ten times. Then, perform the lift with the other arm. Use very light weights at first and gradually increase as necessary.

Flexion of Forearm (Back)

Standing, grasp a weighted bar or hammer, with the weighted end behind you. Flex your wrist by lifting the weight toward the ceiling without moving the arm, exhaling on the work phase. Hold for two seconds, and return to the starting position. Repeat ten times. Then, perform the lift with the other arm. Use very light weights at first and gradually increase as necessary.

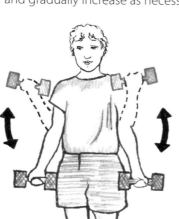

Biceps Curls

Stand with your arms at your sides, palms facing forward and holding light dumbbells. Slowly bend your elbows, bringing the weights toward your shoulders and exhaling. Hold for two seconds and return to the starting position. Repeat ten times. Add more weight as necessary.

Massage Techniques for the Arm

These massage techniques can relieve muscle spasm and pain, increase circulation, and promote the healing of arm injuries.

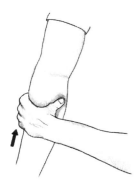

Gliding Self-Massage

With one arm extended, the opposite arm "cups" the extended arm and glides upward. Exhale on the gliding stroke. Repeat as necessary. This gliding massage can also be done on a slightly flexed arm. You can apply friction by pressing the thumb firmly into the muscle and making small side-to-side motions.

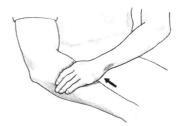

Assisted Gliding Massage

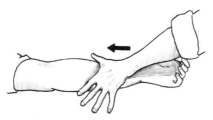

Begin with your arm slightly flexed and resting gently on a solid surface, with your palm facing up. The assisting person uses the palm of his or her hand to glide upward on the arm, with a comfortable amount of pressure. Exhale on the gliding stroke. This massage technique can then be performed with your palm facing down. Repeat as necessary.

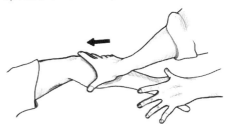

When to Call the Doctor

- If pain persists despite treatment

- If you experience numbness or tingling throughout your arm and elbow

- If there are signs of infection or poor circulation

Questions and Answers

Q: *What are some golf-specific exercises to help in my recovery from golfer's elbow?*

A: It is important to start your recovery process with stretching first. Ice massage is very effective post-workout to help with inflammation of the tendon. Without these two components, your recovery will be compromised.

Use the strengthening exercises for the elbow, shoulder, and wrist that are provided in this book. Try practicing your golf swing lightly with a broomstick in the yard or mimicking your swing in the pool (without the club). Keep your golf game limited to the short game (chipping and putting), then gradually increase your game to full swing. Continued core strengthening of the torso is also critical, as it is always important to maintain a balance in your recovery.

Biomechanics (your body's movement) play a large role in the golf swing. Properly adjusting your golf swing may help take the stress off your elbow. A golf pro at any local golf facility should be able to analyze and properly instruct you on an anatomically correct golf swing.

Q: *I get pain in my upper arm every time I lift something over my head. My job is very physical—what are some things I can do to help myself on the job?*

A: Physical jobs can be troublesome during recovery from an injury. Delivery drivers who lift heavy boxes or carpenters who swing hammers are definitely at a disadvantage. The best advice is make sure to start your day with stretches to warm the shoulders, arms, and wrist (analogous to warming up your car on a cold morning). Continue with some gentle strengthening exercises followed by ice. (Make sure to keep ice handy on the job, as icing throughout the day is very helpful.) At the end of the day, apply gentle massage techniques to keep the muscles supple and supplied with fresh blood for proper healing and nutrition. Some employers will provide an ergonomic analysis of the workplace—check into this or analyze your own ergonomics; that is, analyze your body alignment and make sure that your work space and tools are designed to support proper positioning.

Q: *Is it okay to return to activity with a bruise on my arm?*

A: Resuming activity is fine as long as there is no diminished range of motion, loss of strength, decreased sensation or circulation, or any radiating pain or numbness. We highly recommend icing after activity and applying topical arnica gel to any bruised area (arnica is a homeopathic remedy that can be found in your local health food store).

Prevention Is the Key

- Always warm up with gentle stretching.
- Use proper sporting equipment and techniques.
- Pay attention to any warning signs of injury or pain.
- Always cool down after activity.

WRIST PAIN

Theresa has been a hairstylist for seventeen years. The repetitive motions required to cut and style hair caused severe pain in her wrist and forearm. "I thought I was developing carpal tunnel," says Theresa. "This was very frightening to me because it would affect my ability to work in my occupation." This is what brought her to see me (Kim). I explained how important it was for Theresa to properly stretch her muscles before beginning work. I taught her how to stretch the wrists, shoulders, and neck muscles. She started doing this before work and throughout the day and felt immediate relief from her pain. "I have been stretching every day now and haven't had those types of problems in almost a year," says Theresa.

Wrist pain may be the result of repetitive stress, direct trauma, disease, overuse, or poor mechanics, all of which affect the structure of the soft tissues in the joint, including muscles, tendons, and ligaments. Conditions associated with wrist pain include:

- Carpal tunnel syndrome: entrapment or compression of the median nerve by the surrounding soft tissue/tendons of the wrist

- Wrist ganglion: a fluid-filled cyst located on the outside of the wrist joint, most commonly located on the back of hand

- Wrist tendinitis: inflammation of the tendons surrounding the wrist joint, both on the palm side and back side of wrist; primary cause is overuse

- Wrist sprain or strain: most commonly caused by direct trauma (falling on extended arm) or a forced movement of the wrist without preparation (A sprain involves ligaments and a strain involves the tendons/muscles.)

- Wrist fracture: an injury to the scaphoid (navicular) bone causing severe pain on the thumb side of the wrist (Signs and symptoms include point tenderness, swelling, loss of motion, and possible numbness. *This fracture is serious because it can cause permanent loss of function and strength of the wrist.*)

Sports in which athletes are prone to wrist injuries include baseball, tennis, and golf. Any occupation involving the hands may also lead to wrist injuries—typists, carpenters, massage therapists, and hairdressers are all susceptible to wrist injuries. It is estimated that there were over 500,000 wrist injuries treated in hospitals throughout the United States in 2001. Stretching, exercises to strengthen the wrist, and massage can all help alleviate wrist pain.

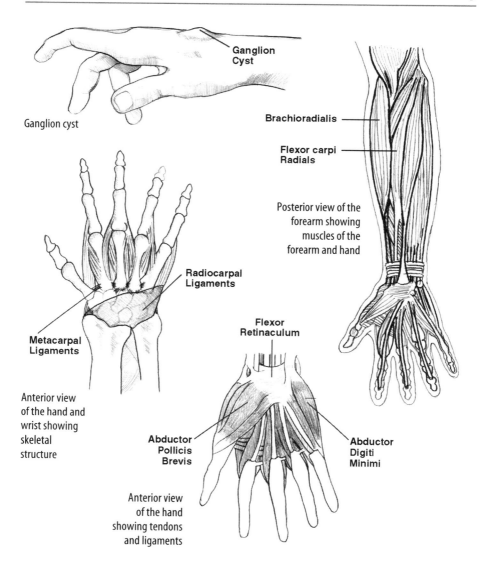

Ganglion Cyst

Ganglion cyst

Brachioradialis

Flexor carpi Radials

Posterior view of the forearm showing muscles of the forearm and hand

Radiocarpal Ligaments

Metacarpal Ligaments

Flexor Retinaculum

Anterior view of the hand and wrist showing skeletal structure

Abductor Pollicis Brevis

Abductor Digiti Minimi

Anterior view of the hand showing tendons and ligaments

FIGURE 6.2. ANATOMY OF THE WRIST

Recipe for a Healthy Wrist

1. Stretch gently, one to two times daily (morning and evening usually works best); do eight to ten repetitions, holding each stretch for two seconds only. Always take your stretch back to the starting position before the next repetition; exhale your breath on the stretch phase.

WRIST PAIN OVERVIEW	
Signs and Symptoms	*Causes*
• Numbness or tingling in the fingers and hand	• Poor ergonomics/mechanics in work space or environment
• Pain in the area surrounding a ganglion cyst	• Overuse injury
• Loss of movement or strength	• Trauma or direct fall on extended arm
• Pain during movement	• Athletic injury
• Swelling, discoloration, or deformity	• Repetitive stress injury (from typing or using a mouse)

2. Follow stretching with strengthening exercises to wrist and forearm. Repeat exercises two to three times weekly, allowing for one day of rest in between.

3. Perform RICHES: rest, ice, compression, heat, elevation, and support (see Chapter 3). In particular, we recommend ice massage to the wrist, two to four times daily for ten minutes each time, using an ice cup or ice pack. Make small circular motions with the ice over the injured or painful area.

4. Make changes to ergonomics or work environment to alleviate any repetitive stress on the wrist (carpal tunnel syndrome). Also, learn to be more aware of your posture and make corrections.

5. Self-massage techniques or assisted techniques can be applied two to three times daily. Massage should not be applied directly to an injury but rather to the surrounding area.

6. When returning to exercise or going to work, warm up chest, shoulders, arms, wrist, and hands first to prepare your body for repetitive stress. Interrupt your day frequently to stretch and correct your posture. If possible, ice two to three times during the day; this reduces the amount of swelling or inflammation that may occur.

7. Maintain a proper diet and hydration for recovery (see Chapter 2).

Stretches for the Wrist

A number of stretches have proven effective in promoting flexibility and alleviating wrist pain.

Forearm/Wrist Extension I

Hold your right arm out straight with the palm facing up. Grip the fingers of your right hand with your other hand and gently bend them downward and back. Hold for two seconds, exhaling on the stretch phase, and return to the starting position. Repeat eight to ten times. Then, perform the stretch on the left arm.

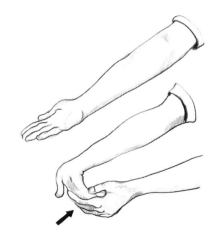

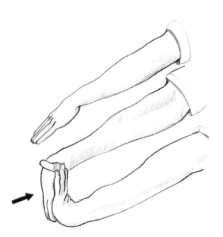

Forearm/Wrist Extension II

Hold your left arm out straight with the palm facing down. Extend the fingers up and back, assisting with your other hand to gently bend the palm and fingers of the left hand. Hold for two seconds, exhaling on the stretch phase, and return to the starting position. Repeat eight to ten times. Then, perform the stretch on the right arm.

Forearm/Wrist Flexion I

Hold your left arm out straight with the palm facing down. Flex the wrist downward, assisting with your other hand to gently bend the left wrist. Hold for two seconds, exhaling on the stretch phase, and return to starting position. Repeat eight to ten times. Then, perform the stretch on the right arm.

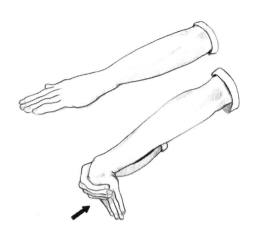

Forearm/Wrist Flexion II

Hold your left arm out straight and make a fist. Flex the wrist downward, assisting with your other hand to gently bend the left wrist. Hold for two seconds, exhaling on the stretch phase, and return to the starting position. Repeat eight to ten times. Then, perform the stretch on the right arm.

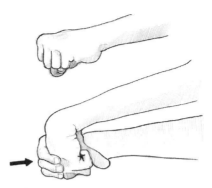

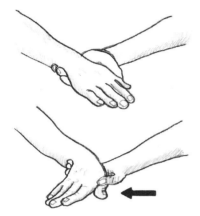

Ulnar Flexion

Hold out your right arm in front of you, keeping the elbow extended and the palm facing downward. Use your other hand as shown and flex the wrist gently toward the little-finger side. Hold for two seconds, exhaling on the stretch phase, and return to the starting position. Repeat eight to ten times. Then, perform the stretch on the left arm.

Radial Flexion

Hold out your right arm in front of you, keeping the elbow extended and the palm facing down. Use your other hand as shown and flex the wrist gently toward the thumb side. Hold for two seconds, exhaling on the stretch phase, and return to the starting position. Repeat eight to ten times. Then, perform the stretch on the other arm.

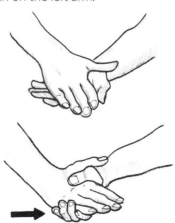

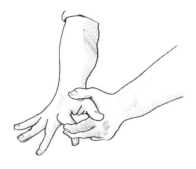

Finger Flexion

Using the opposite hand, extend each finger, one at a time, downward as far as possible. Hold for two seconds, exhaling on the stretch phase, before moving to the next finger. Repeat eight to ten times. Then, perform the stretch on the other hand.

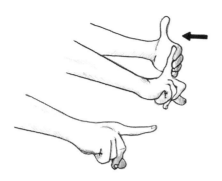

Finger Extension I

Extend your wrist back and, using the opposite hand, flex each finger, one at a time, backward as far as possible. (Help yourself by assisting with the entire finger, not just the fingertip; also note that this exercise can be done with the elbow straight or bent.) Hold for two seconds, exhaling on the stretch phase, before moving to the next finger. Repeat eight to ten times. Then, perform the stretch on the other hand.

Finger Extension II

With your palm facing up, flex each finger, one at a time, backward as far as possible, using the opposite hand. (Help yourself by assisting with the entire finger, not just the fingertip.) Hold for two seconds, exhaling on the stretch phase, before moving to the next finger. Repeat eight to ten times. Then, perform the stretch on the other hand.

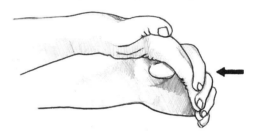

Exercises for the Wrist

The following exercises will help you condition your wrist muscles and recover from injury.

Wrist Roller

Use a weight tied with rope to a wood dowel or shortened broomstick. Holding the dowel in your hands, extend your arms straight in front of you at shoulder level and use your wrists to wind the rope around the dowel, lifting the weight. Be sure to use each wrist's full range of motion. Then, use the wrists to roll the weight back down. Exhale your breath on the work phase. Repeat three to five times. Start with a light weight and increase as necessary.

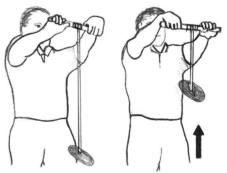

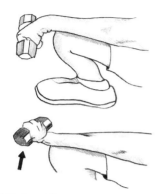

Wrist Extension

Support your arm on the thigh, palm facing down and holding a light dumbbell. Extend the wrist up and back as far as it will go. Keep your grip as relaxed as possible, and exhale on the work phase. Return to starting position. Repeat fifteen times. Then, perform the lift with the other arm. Add more weight as necessary.

Wrist Flexion

Support your arm on the thigh, palm facing up and holding a light dumbbell. Start with your grip relaxed and hand hanging down over your knee. Flex your wrist toward you as far as it will go, exhaling on the work phase. Return to starting position. Repeat fifteen times. Then, perform the lift with the other arm. Add more weight as necessary.

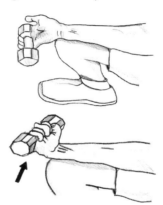

Flexion of Forearm (Front)

Standing, grasp a weighted bar or hammer, with the weighted end in front of you. Flex your wrist by lifting the weight toward the ceiling without moving the arm, exhaling on the work phase. Return to starting position. Repeat ten times. Then, perform the lift with the other arm. Start with a light weight and increase as necessary.

Extension of Forearm (Back)

Standing, grasp a weighted bar or hammer, with the weighted end behind you. Flex your wrist by lifting the weight toward the ceiling without moving the arm, exhaling on the work phase. Return to starting position. Repeat ten times. Repeat the lift with the other arm. Start with a light weight and increase as necessary.

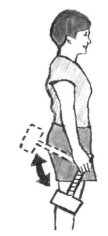

Pronation of the Wrist

Lie on your right side, with your right elbow bent and held against your body. Grasp a weighted bar (wood dowel with a weight, or a hammer) in your right hand, with your thumb pointed down. Rotate your hand until the weight and your thumb point up. Exhale on the work phase, and return to the starting position. Repeat fifteen times. Then perform the lift on your left side. Start with a light weight and add increase as necessary.

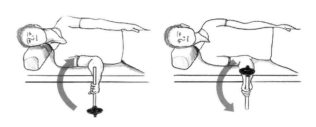

Supination of the Wrist

Lie on your right side, with your right elbow bent and held against your body. Grasp a weighted bar (wood dowel with a weight or a hammer) in your right hand, with your thumb pointed up. Rotate your hand until the weight points up and your thumb points down. Exhale on the work phase, and return to the starting position. Repeat fifteen times. Then perform the lift on your left side. Start with a light weight and increase as necessary.

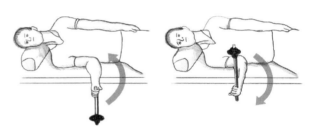

Massage Techniques for the Wrist/Forearm

These massage techniques can relieve muscle spasm and pain, increase circulation, and promote the healing of wrist injuries.

Gliding Self-Massage

With one arm extended, the opposite arm "cups" the extended arm and glides upward. Exhale on the gliding stroke. Repeat as necessary. This gliding massage can also be done on a slightly flexed arm. You can apply friction by pressing the thumb firmly into the muscle and making small side-to-

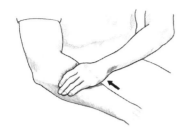

side motions. Note that massage to the arm is important to alleviate tension and strain on the wrist joint; wrist muscles attach at the elbow, run through the wrist joint and attach at the end of the fingertips.

Assisted Gliding Massage

Begin with your arm slightly flexed and resting gently on a solid surface, with your palm facing up. The assisting person uses

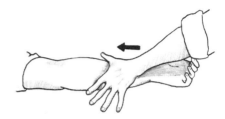

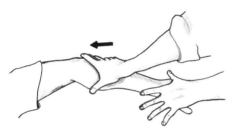

the palm of his or her hand to glide upward on the arm, with a comfortable amount of pressure. Exhale on the gliding stroke. This massage technique can then be performed with your palm facing down. Repeat as necessary.

When to Call the Doctor

• If pain persists despite treatment

• If numbing or tingling in the wrist persists or worsens

• If you have poor circulation or deformity

Carpal Tunnel Syndrome

Don't get "tunnel vision." Carpal tunnel syndrome does not necessarily originate at the wrist—it can also start at the neck and shoulders. Be sure to include neck and shoulder stretches as part of your recovery from carpal tunnel (see Chapter 4).

Questions and Answers

Q: *Should I wear a wrist brace?*

A: Yes, if recommended by your healthcare professional or if it is necessary to take pressure off of soft tissues (muscles, tendons, ligaments) or bone structure. If no broken bones are present, remove the brace and gently do stretching exercises several times throughout the day. Follow with ice treatment. Always follow the advice of your healthcare professional.

> **Q:** *With a sprained/strained wrist, should I use heat?*
>
> **A:** In the acute phase (sudden onset), or during the first seventy-two hours, use ice therapy only. After the first seventy-two hours, and if there is no swelling present, heat may be applied (or hot-and-cold contrast applications). If the condition worsens, see your healthcare practitioner.
>
> **Q:** *Should I "pop" my ganglion cyst?*
>
> **A:** No. Consult your healthcare professional so that the cyst may be drained (or surgically removed in severe cases). By trying to "pop" it, trauma may occur, causing possible damage to the wrist.

Prevention Is the Key

- Use correct ergonomics; that is, make sure your body alignment is correct and that your home and work space and tools are designed to support this alignment. If you are unsure of your positioning, have a biomechanical assessment done to help you.

- Start each day with stretches, being careful to maintain good muscle balance and to stretch both sides.

- Get proper nutrition and hydration during recovery.

- Be aware of your spinal posture while seated and standing; correct any imbalances.

- End each day with a cooling-down process. Stretch lightly to allow for proper blood flow to tired and fatigued muscles. This helps to circulate fresh oxygenated blood throughout your body.

- Relax and practice deep breathing and positive affirmations.

- Use proper equipment and correct technique when returning to exercise.

HAND PAIN

Hand pain may be the result of direct trauma, injury, or disease affecting the skeletal structure of the hand or the muscles surrounding the wrist joint. Conditions associated with hand pain include:

- Hand bruise: discoloration to the soft tissues of the hand, due to direct trauma

- Arthritis: disease that causes inflammation in the bones and joints; can lead to deformity

- "Jammed" finger: direct trauma at the end of the finger that can cause damage to the finger joints or a broken finger

- Hand sprain, strain, or tendinitis: inflammation of the muscles, ligaments, and tendons of the hand; often due to violent overstretching or overuse of the hand

Hand pain or injury is common in basketball (jamming of the fingers), football, and in types of work that rely on extensive use of the hands—artists, massage therapists, carpenters, floor installers, hairdressers, and typists are susceptible to hand pain or injury. There are approximately 490,000 cases of hand injuries per year in the United States.

Stretching, exercises to strengthen the hand muscles, and massage can all help alleviate hand pain.

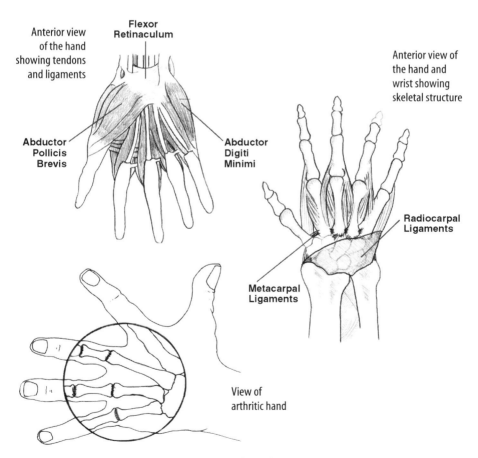

FIGURE 6.3. ANATOMY OF THE HAND

HAND PAIN OVERVIEW	
Signs and Symptoms	*Causes*
• Pain at the time of injury	• Direct trauma
• Swelling or discoloration	• Overuse or repetitive stress
• Decrease in movement or function	• Violent or excessive movement
• Point tenderness and possible numbness	• Lack of lubricant (synovial fluid) in the joints
• Constant localized or radiating pain due to systemic disease (arthritis)	• Stretched tendons and ligaments

Recipe for a Healthy Hand

1. Stretch one to two times daily. It is important to warm up the forearm and wrist prior to stretching your fingers, as this will increase the blood flow throughout the region. Do eight to ten repetitions, holding each stretch for two seconds only. Always take your stretch back to the starting position before the next repetition; exhale your breath on the stretch phase. Also, be sure to stretch gently before beginning to work, particularly in jobs involving heavy use of the wrists and hands. If you have an injury, it is best to ice for ten minutes before stretching. For arthritic patients, heat applied before stretching or other activity may help stimulate blood flow to the area.

2. Perform RICHES: rest, ice, compression, heat, elevation, and support (see Chapter 3).

3. Do strengthening exercises three times weekly, with one day of rest in between; always stretch before you strengthen. One easy way to strengthen the hand and wrist is to keep a "squishy" ball with you at all times—squeeze it for a few minutes to strengthen and reduce stress.

4. Ice affected area for ten to fifteen minutes after activity; ice packs or ice massage are most effective (unless you have ice sensitivity). Cold ice baths are also effective: fill a small bucket or one side of the kitchen sink with cold water and add ice; soak hand and wrist in the ice water for several minutes.

5. Fix your work area to be ergonomically correct. Be aware of your posture, sit up straight, and properly position your keyboard. In labor-intensive jobs, always protect your hands.

6. Self-massage techniques can be used one to two times daily.

7. When returning to exercise, always take time to warm up properly, and cool down with additional stretching and ice after activity.

8. Maintain a proper diet and hydration for recovery (see Chapter 2).

Stretches for the Hand

A number of stretches have proven effective in promoting flexibility and alleviating hand pain.

Finger Flexion

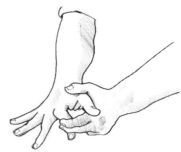

Using the opposite hand, extend each finger, one at a time, downward as far as possible. Hold for two seconds, exhaling on the stretch phase, before moving to the next finger. Repeat eight to ten times. Then, perform the stretch on the other hand.

Finger Extension I

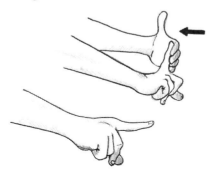

Extend your wrist back and, using the opposite hand, flex each finger, one at a time, backward as far as possible. (Help yourself by assisting with the entire finger, not just the fingertip; also note that this exercise can be done with the elbow straight or bent.) Hold for two seconds, exhaling on the stretch phase, before moving to the next finger. Repeat eight to ten times. Then, perform the stretch on the other hand.

Finger Extension II

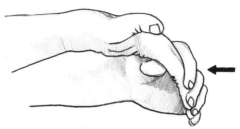

With your palm facing up, flex each finger, one at a time, backward as far as possible, using the opposite hand. (Help yourself by assisting with the entire finger, not just the fingertip.) Hold for two seconds, exhaling on the stretch phase, before moving to the next finger. Repeat eight to ten times. Then, perform the stretch on the other hand.

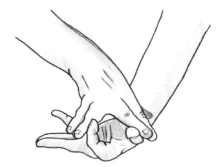

Finger Abduction

Using the thumb and index finger of your left hand, gently spread each pair of fingers on your right hand. Hold for two seconds, exhaling on the stretch phase, and return to the starting position. Repeat eight to ten times. Then, perform the stretch on the left hand.

Thumb Stretch

With your right palm facing up, use your left hand to stretch the right thumb away from the rest of the hand. Hold for two seconds, exhaling on the stretch phase, and return to the starting position. Repeat eight to ten times. Then, perform the stretch on your left hand.

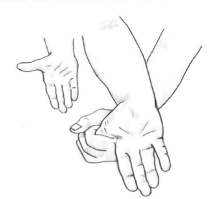

Exercises for the Hand

The following exercises will help you condition your hand muscles and recover from injury.

Finger Extensor Exercise

Place a rubber band around your thumb and fingers, then slowly move them away from the center of the hand, pushing out against the rubber band. Slowly return to the starting position. Repeat ten times with each hand. Use smaller rubber bands for more resistance, as needed.

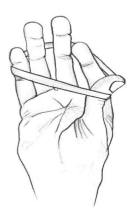

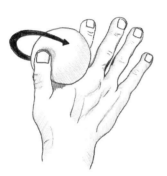

Thumb Adduction

Place a rubber ball between your thumb and forefinger. Use your thumb to roll the ball over the top of the index finger. Relax. Repeat ten times with each hand.

Grip Strengthening

Squeeze a rubber ball in your hand without using the thumb. Relax. Repeat ten times with each hand. Make sure, as you allow the ball to flex back to its normal position after squeezing, that you release your grip in a slow and controlled movement.

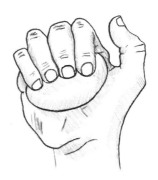

Massage Techniques for the Hand

These massage techniques can relieve muscle spasm and pain, increase circulation, and promote the healing of hand injuries.

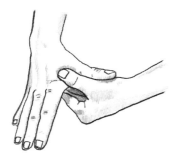

Trigger-Point Massage in Web of Thumb

Using your thumb and index finger, gently compress the area between the thumb and index finger of the opposite hand. Hold for thirty seconds and then relax. Repeat on the other hand. (This technique can also help relieve headaches.)

Stripping Massage in the Palm

Rest your hand on your thigh, palm facing up. With the opposite thumb, start pressing at the base of the palm and glide toward the fingers. Repeat as necessary.

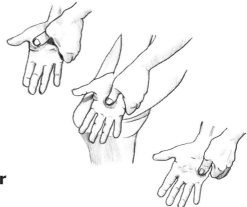

When to Call the Doctor

- If pain persists despite treatment
- If you have a lack of circulation or deformity
- If you feel numbness and tingling in the hand
- If there is continued swelling, discoloration, or loss of function

Questions and Answers

Q: *Is it dangerous to "pop" my knuckles?*

A: Medically, popping your knuckles is merely a release of pressure within the joint. Once the pressure is released within the joint, it can be easier to stretch and increase range of motion in the fingers. However, it is not recommended that you forcefully pop your knuckles, because you could damage soft-tissue structures.

Q: *How soon can I return to activity after a strain to the muscles in my hand?*

A: You may gradually return to activity once you have met the following conditions:

Clearance by your physician

Signs and symptoms have decreased

Strength and mobility have increased (compare to other hand)

Q: *What is the best way to treat a "jammed" finger?*

A: The best treatment for a jammed finger is to ice it immediately, followed by a range of gentle motion exercises. If no swelling is present, apply heat to aid in stretching and warm-up activities. You may "buddy tape" your finger for additional support (see Figure 6.4).

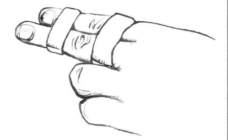

If the injury is severe, consult your physician and immobilize the finger by buddy taping or splinting it. Jamming injuries to the thumb should be referred to a physician.

FIGURE 6.4. Buddy taping for an injured finger

Prevention Is the Key

• Start out with proper warm-up exercises and stretching.

• Remove all jewelry during activity—rings and watches can snag and cause swelling and serious damage to the hands and fingers.

• Cool down properly—stretching and icing following activity.

• Keep fingernails and hands clean and neatly manicured; this will help decrease the chances of injuries and infection.

Chapter 7

Hip and Low-Back Pain

Kate had been an active runner, cyclist, swimmer, hiker, and rower for years and thrived on activity as an antidote to her sedentary office job. But over the years, musculoskeletal imbalances began to take their toll and intense hip/sciatic nerve pain forced her to quit running and other high-impact activities in her late twenties. She had multiple MRIs (magnetic resonance imaging) and tried chiropractic treatments, anti-inflammatory medications, and physical therapy, but to no avail. "I never realized how the types of exercises and stretches I was doing were probably causing more harm than good," Kate says. She then met Kim and began learning the Active Isolated Stretching method, which has made a tremendous difference. This past summer, at the age of forty-seven, she even won a road-cycling championship. Kate sticks with her stretching routine and it helps her through periodic flare-ups. "After living with chronic pain for many years, and trying many conventional and alternative therapies, I feel at peace knowing I have a tool for self-healing."

HIP PAIN

Hip pain may be the result of inflammation, poor biomechanics (body movement), disease, direct trauma, or overuse of the joint and the surrounding soft tissues. Conditions associated with hip pain include:

- Hip bursitis: inflammation of the fluid-filled sac on the side of the hip

- Iliotibial band syndrome (ITBS): inflammation of the thick band of tissue that originates at the hip and attaches to the outside of the knee

- "Snapping hip": clicking in the hip joint due to forced range of motion, causing pain and inflammation in the joint; usually seen in young female gymnasts and dancers

- Hip pointer: bruise to the iliac crest (top) of the hip due to direct trauma and characterized by localized pain, discoloration, and possible temporary paralysis

- Hip strain, sprain, or tendinitis: injury and inflammation of the muscles, tendons, and ligaments of the hip

Hip pain may be caused by activities that involve repetitive pounding of the joint, such as running and jumping, or by sports that may involve direct trauma, such

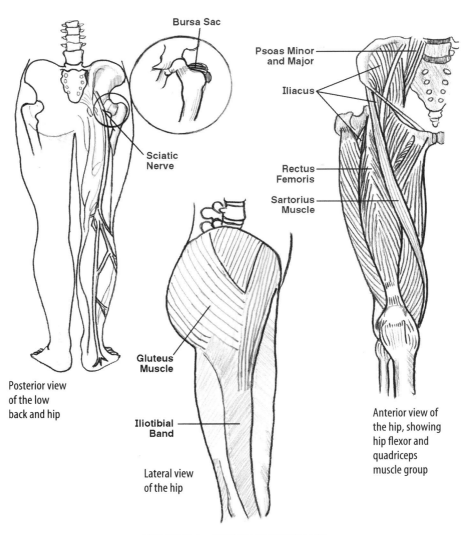

FIGURE 7.1. ANATOMY OF THE HIP

HIP PAIN OVERVIEW

Signs and Symptoms

- Pain in the hip while sitting still or moving
- Clicking sound when moving hip
- Tenderness or swelling
- Loss of function, limping, or inability to walk
- Loss of strength
- Discoloration
- Numbness and tingling throughout hip, low back, and buttocks
- Radiating or referred pain (in buttocks, outside of knee, or in hip)

Causes

- Injury due to direct trauma or overuse
- Arthritic disease causing inflammation in the hip joint and bursae
- Excessive, forced range of motion (dancing, gymnastics)
- Excessive weight-bearing activity due to obesity
- Tightness in the muscles in the back of the leg, buttocks, and low back
- Poor body mechanics (genetic deformity, bow-legged, knock-kneed, wide hips in women)

as football or rugby. Hip fractures are prevalent among the elderly due to falls; hip injuries may result from degeneration or overuse.

Stretching, exercises to strengthen the hip muscles, and massage can all help alleviate hip pain.

Recipe for a Healthy Hip

1. Stretch gently one to two times daily; do eight to ten repetitions, holding each stretch for two seconds only. Always take the stretch back to the starting position before the next repetition; exhale your breath on the stretch phase.

2. Follow stretching with strengthening exercises three times weekly, with one day of rest in between.

3. Ice two to four times daily for ten minutes each time, using an ice pack. Contrast applications, alternating heat (moist heat preferred) and ice, are beneficial if no signs of swelling are present—but only after seventy-two hours have passed since the injury. Perform contrast therapy by applying ice for three minutes, then heat for two minutes, and repeating the cycle two to three times, ending with ice. This therapy can be used several times per day.

4. Consider chiropractic care or consult a podiatrist (foot doctor) for shoe inserts that support your arch and foot.

5. Massage techniques can be applied one to two times daily.

6. When returning to exercise, warm up properly, gradually increase exercise intensity, and cool down with stretching and ice after activity.

7. Maintain a proper diet and hydration for recovery (see Chapter 2). Be sure to balance food intake with level of activity to avoid excessive weight gain.

Stretches for the Hip

A number of stretches have proven effective in promoting flexibility and alleviating hip pain.

Single-Leg Pelvic Tilt

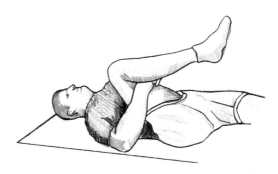

Lie on your back and flex your right leg, leaving the left leg extended (if you have a sore back, the left leg can be flexed). Holding the right leg under the thigh, pull it toward your right shoulder (not the chest), contracting the stomach and hip-flexor muscles. Exhale on the stretch phase and hold for two seconds, then return to the starting position. Repeat eight to ten times. Then, perform the same stretch with the left leg.

Gluteal Stretch

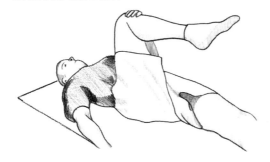

Lie on your back and bend your right knee to a 90-degree angle. Grab that knee with your left hand and move it across your body toward the left shoulder. The left leg stays extended, moves toward the midline of the body, and rotates internally. Exhale on the stretch phase and hold for two seconds, then return to the starting position. Repeat eight to ten times. Then, perform the same stretch with the left knee.

Hamstring Stretch (Bent Knee)

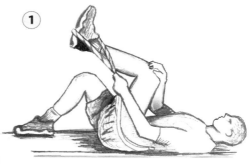

Lie on your back with both knees bent and feet resting flat on the floor. Lift your left leg, keeping the knee bent, and wrap a rope under the ball of the foot. From

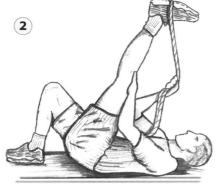

the bent position, extend your knee straight up, using the rope for assistance. The right leg remains with knee bent and foot flat on the floor. Exhale on the stretch phase and hold for two seconds, then return to the starting position. Repeat eight to ten times. Then, perform the same stretch with the right leg.

Hamstring Stretch (Straight Leg)

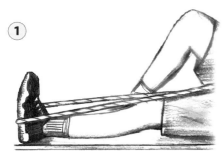

Lie on your back. Your right leg is bent with the foot flat on the floor; your left leg is straight with a rope wrapped around the ball of the foot. Contract

the quadriceps muscle (front of thigh) of the left leg, keeping the knee extended, and lift straight up toward the ceiling. Use the rope to assist the stretch, not to help lift the leg. Exhale on the stretch phase and hold for two seconds, then return to the starting position. Repeat eight to ten times. Then, perform the same stretch with the right leg.

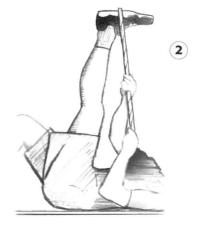

Groin Stretch

Lie on your back with legs extended, and wrap a rope under the ball of your right foot and toward the inside of the ankle. The uninvolved (left) leg should be moved slightly away from the body. Using the hip muscles, move the right leg away from the middle of the body, using the rope for assistance. Keep your toes pointed toward the ceiling as the leg slides along the floor. Avoid lifting

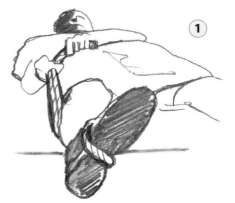

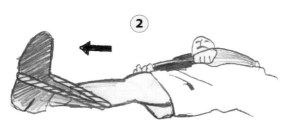

the leg during the stretch. Exhale on the stretch phase and hold for two seconds, then return to the starting position. Repeat eight to ten times. Then, perform the same stretch with the left leg.

Iliotibial Band/Hip Abductor Stretch I

Lie on your back and wrap a rope under the ball of your left foot and to the outside of the ankle. Keep both legs extended and rotate the right leg slightly inward and toward the midline

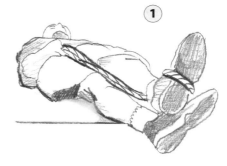

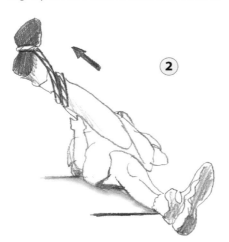

of the body. Rotate the left leg slightly outward, with the toes pointed outward. Keeping the knee extended and using the rope for assistance, move the left leg across the body to the right. Exhale on the stretch phase and hold for two seconds, then return to the starting position. Repeat eight to ten times. Then, perform the same stretch with the right leg.

Iliotibial Band/Hip Abductor Stretch II

Building on Stretch I above, this stretch involves more of the hip muscle (gluteal medius). Lie on your back and wrap the rope under the ball of your right foot and to the inside of the ankle. Keep both legs straight with your left leg turned slightly inward and moved toward

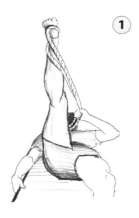

the midline of the body. Lift the right leg up until you have reached a 90-degree angle at the hip, then move the leg directly across the body (toward the left). Keep your knee extended. Exhale on the stretch phase and hold for two seconds, then return to the starting position. Repeat eight to ten times. Then, perform the same stretch with the left leg.

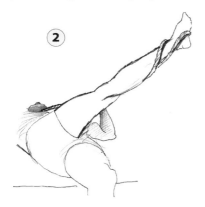

Hip Flexor

Kneel with your right knee on the floor (place a pad under the knee). Your left leg is bent at the knee with your foot flat on the ground about twelve inches in front of the left knee. Lean forward (contract your gluteal muscle through the movement) onto the flexed (left) knee until the knee is directly above your left ankle. If your knee moves in front of the ankle, move the foot forward. Contract your stomach muscles as you do this

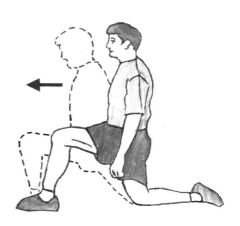

movement. Exhale on the stretch phase and hold for two seconds, then return to the starting position. Repeat eight to ten times. Then, perform the same stretch with the left knee on the floor and the right knee extended.

Exercises for the Hip

The following exercises will help you condition your hip muscles and recover from injury.

Straight-Leg Raise

Lie on your back with the left leg bent and relaxed. With the right leg extended, lift the leg slowly, keeping the foot flexed and toes pointed toward your chest. Exhale on the work phase, then slowly return to the starting position. Repeat ten times. Then, perform the same exercise with the left leg. You can add an ankle weight for more resistance as needed.

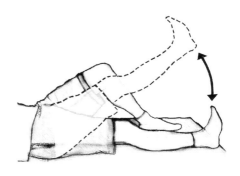

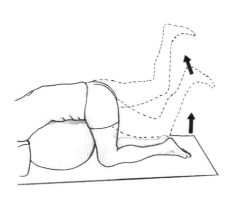

Gluteal Strengthening on Stability Ball

Lie forward on an exercise ball, relax your upper body, and begin with both knees on the floor. Keeping the knee flexed, lift the right leg toward the ceiling. Exhale on the work phase, then slowly return to the starting position. Repeat fifteen times. Then, perform the same exercise with the left leg. You can add an ankle weight for more resistance as needed.

Side Leg Raise for the Hips

Lie on your side with both legs extended. Lift the top leg toward the ceiling with the knee extended and foot flexed (toes pointed toward the chest). Rotate the leg slightly inward so that the heel is higher than the toes. The resting leg can be straight or slightly bent. Exhale on the work phase, then slowly return to the starting position. Repeat ten times. Then, perform the same exercise with the other leg. Add an ankle weight for more resistance as needed.

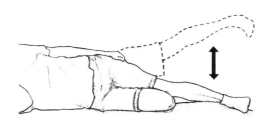

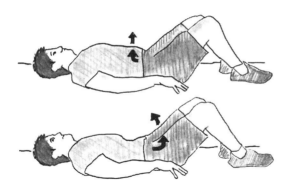

Pelvic Tilt

Lie on your back with both legs flexed and feet flat on the floor. Tilt your pelvis up and back while contracting the lower abdominal muscles. Your pelvis should be lifted slightly at the end of the movement. Exhale on the work phase and hold for three to five seconds, then return to the starting position. Repeat ten times. Place small weights on the abdomen for resistance as needed.

Groin (Adductor) Strengthening Exercise

Lie on your side on the floor. The left leg is extended and resting on the seat of a chair (or a bench). The right leg is underneath the chair, with knee extended and toes flexed toward the chest. Lift the right leg toward the chair, being sure to

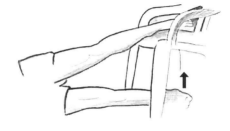

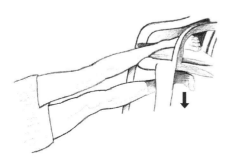

keep the toes flexed. Keep your stomach muscles slightly tightened. Exhale on the work phase, then slowly return to the starting position. Repeat ten times. Then, perform the same exercise with the left leg. Add an ankle weight for more resistance as needed.

Hip Exercise Tip

We recommend non-gravitational exercises, such as water aerobics, water jogging, and swimming, for individuals with hip replacements or severe hip conditions (arthritis or balance disorders). You will receive the benefits of exercise without pounding or irritating the hip joint. Water allows for sixteen times more resistance than air.

Massage Techniques for the Hip

These massage techniques can relieve muscle spasm and pain, increase circulation, and promote the healing of hip injuries.

Gliding Iliotibial-Band Massage

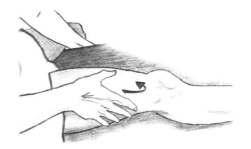

Sit with your leg extended. Stroke the leg from the thigh down toward the foot, using long, circular movements. Repeat as necessary.

Assisted Gliding Iliotibial-Band Massage

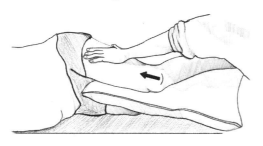

Lie on your side with a pillow between your knees. The massage assistant will use the palm of his or her hand to gently glide along the iliotibial band, starting at the knee and working up the thigh. Exhale during the gliding phase. Repeat as necessary.

When to Call the Doctor

• If pain persists despite treatment

• If you feel constant numbness or tingling

• If walking or standing is painful

• If you experience continued swelling

• If you have continued loss of strength or function

Questions and Answers

Q: *What are some alternatives to running on pavement in order to help alleviate pain in my hip and knee?*

A: If you are running on the road, change the side of the road you are running on according to the angle of the road (make sure you do this safely, watching out for traffic). Consider changing to softer surfaces, such as grass, rubberized track, dirt, or a good-quality treadmill. You may want to alternate your exercise surfaces: Monday on a treadmill, Tuesday in the pool (water jogging), Wednesday on grass, Thursday on a dirt trail, and so on. Be sure to include a rest day.

Q: *Is it safe to combine different therapies/treatments for my hip?*

A: Yes, we recommend that the following healthcare professionals assist in the treatment of a hip injury: orthopedic doctor (specializes in bones and joints), massage therapist, physical therapist, chiropractor, acupuncturist, and podiatrist (for shoe inserts to help with biomechanics of the hip). Remember, this list can be expanded.

Prevention Is the Key

- Wear good shoes that provide proper support and cushion for your feet.

- Practice daily stretching and movement.

- Run or jog on good surfaces.

- Avoid sitting down for extended periods of time. Even on an airplane you can walk the aisles—if you are traveling long distances, walk and stretch every couple of hours.

- Always stretch before you go to bed to ease built-up tension in the muscles, tendons, and ligaments.

LOW-BACK PAIN

Connie was diagnosed with sciatica due to decreased disk space in her spine. After medication and physical therapy reduced the back pain to a tolerable level, she had decided that this was something she would just have to live with. But while looking for a massage therapist for her husband, Connie decided to try massage herself and that's how I (Kim) came to know her. I taught her some stretching techniques for her back and, as we worked together, the episodes of back pain occurred less and less frequently. "Better yet, Kim taught me what to do for myself when I am stiff and sore," says Connie, "and this knowledge has finally chased the back pain away."

Over 80 percent of Americans suffer from back pain. Low-back pain may be the result of direct trauma, violent twisting, or overstretching of soft tissues of the low back, including ligaments, tendons, and muscles. Damage may occur to the ligaments that attach to the disk and sacroiliac joint. Poor posture (from genetic and structural problems) may result in injury to the muscles or tendons that attach to the low back (lumbar disk). Conditions associated with low-back pain include:

- Herniated or "slipped" disk: when the ligaments supporting the disk experience a tear, thereby exposing the "jelly" (contents) of the inner vertebral disk; commonly takes place toward the rear of the disk, sometimes affecting the nerves

- Lumbar (lower back) sprain or strain: injury to the soft tissue (muscle, tendons, or ligaments) of the lumbar spine

- Thoracic (middle back) sprain or strain: injury to the soft tissue (muscle, tendons, or ligaments) of the middle back (pain may start in the middle back and travel down toward the lower back)

- Sciatica: pain along the sciatic nerve, the largest nerve in the body, originating at the lower lumbar spine and running through the pelvis and down both legs; may result from a herniated lumbar disk or sacral disk, or from a dislocation of the sacroiliac joint (Muscle spasms in the buttocks can also cause some sciatic nerve pain or radiating pain down either leg.)

Low-back pain can also be the result of conditions of poor structural posture, such as lordosis (swayback), scoliosis (lateral curvature of the spine or S curve), and kyphosis (hunchback). See Figure 7.2 for an illustration of postural deficiencies. These postures can result in nerve pain or nerve dysfunction, pain, tightness, or spasm in muscles surrounding the skeletal structures, and possible muscle weakness and imbalance.

LOW-BACK PAIN OVERVIEW

Signs and Symptoms	*Causes*
• Severe pain in the low back	• Weakness of fluid inside of a disk
• Weakness and numbness (shooting pains down the leg)	• Obesity
• Tenderness in the low back	• Improper lifting or stressful activity
• A "popping" or tearing feeling	• Muscular imbalances
• Swelling in the low back	• Direct force on ligaments
• Pain with movement	• Overstretching or overexertion
• Loss of strength	• Growing older
• Pain when sneezing	

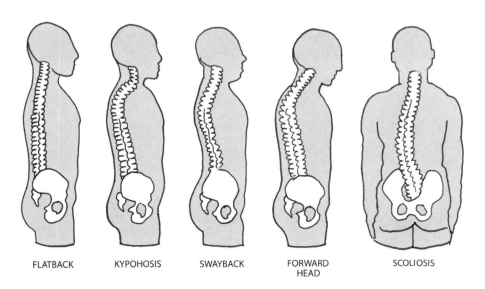

FLATBACK   KYPOHOSIS   SWAYBACK   FORWARD HEAD   SCOLIOSIS

FIGURE 7.2. POSTURAL DEFICIENCIES (Identify your spine in this picture.)

We recommend a complete flexibility program for these conditions followed by overall muscle strengthening. The stretches in this chapter and in Chapter 8 on the upper leg and knee illustrate some of the stretches that can be used to help these conditions. They were particularly helpful for Miriam, one of Kim's clients. Miriam had been searching for solutions to surgery for scoliosis since 1998. "After having searched for twelve years to find solutions—real ones, not empty promises—to my pain from scoliosis," says Miriam, "I finally found Kim, who introduced me to Active Isolated Stretching."

While several methods gave her hope and some improvement, Active Isolated Stretching was something she could easily do at home and gave her relief within minutes, not months or years. "Understanding the process makes me want to stick with it completely," says Miriam. "Thank goodness, because I was wondering when I was ever going to feel like a normal human being again." Your healthcare professional may offer further recommendations regarding protocols for lordosis, scoliosis, and kyphosis.

Any sport can irritate the lower back, particularly golf (90 percent of golf injuries involve the lower back), football, soccer, basketball, swimming, running, and cycling. Low-back pain can also be the result of muscle, nerve, disk, and bone/joint pathologies.

Stretching, exercises to strengthen the low-back muscles, and massage can all help alleviate low-back pain.

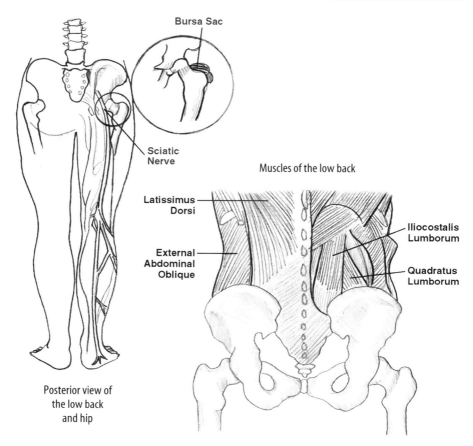

FIGURE 7.3. ANATOMY OF THE LOW BACK

Recipe for a Healthy Low Back

1. Start each day with stretching to prepare the muscles for the day's activities. Hold each stretch for two seconds and return to the starting position between each stretch. Repeat eight to ten times; exhale your breath on the stretch phase.

2. Do strengthening exercises two to three times weekly, allowing one day of rest in between and beginning with light weights. Strengthening is critically important to help achieve a proper balance. Always stretch before you strengthen.

3. Use ice packs or ice bags to reduce pain and swelling. Apply ice two to four times daily for ten minutes each time, especially after stretching or strengthening. Heat (moist heat is preferred) can be used for non-acute pain and usually works best for sciatic nerve problems.

4. Use proper ergonomics when lifting heavy objects (see "Proper Ergonomics for Lifting Heavy Objects" below).

5. Consider consulting a podiatrist (foot doctor) for shoe inserts that support your arch and foot.

6. Massage techniques can be applied one to two times daily. Professional massage is helpful several times a week for chronic low-back pain.

7. Start exercising regularly. When returning to exercise, warm up properly, gradually increase your intensity, and finish with a cool down involving stretching followed by an ice application.

8. Maintain a proper diet and hydration for recovery (see Chapter 2).

9. Achieve and maintain a balance of flexibility and strength throughout the entire torso, low back, and leg areas. Other modalities or therapies can be helpful in relieving low-back pain, such as chiropractic, physical therapy, massage therapy, acupuncture, and Active Isolated Stretching (the Mattes Method). It is advisable in severe chronic conditions to seek the advice of your physician before exercise or treatment therapies. X-rays and MRIs are commonly used to identify problems and guide your healing protocol.

Proper Ergonomics for Lifting Heavy Objects

- When picking something up, tighten your stomach muscles, bend your knees into a half-squat position, and keep your back as straight as possible.

- When lifting, keep your back straight and your stomach muscles tightened, and lift with your legs.

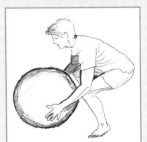 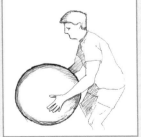 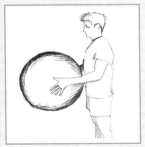

Note: If you can't lift comfortably with your legs, then the object is too heavy and you need to get some help.

Stretches for the Low Back

A number of stretches have proven effective in promoting flexibility and alleviating low-back pain.

Single-Leg Pelvic Tilt

Lie on your back and flex your right leg, leaving the left leg extended (if you have a sore back, the left leg can be flexed). Holding the right leg under the thigh, pull it toward your right shoulder (not the chest), contracting the stomach and hip-flexor muscles. Exhale on the stretch phase and hold for two seconds, then return to the starting position. Repeat eight to ten times. Then, perform the same stretch with the left leg.

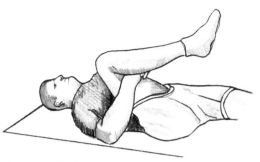

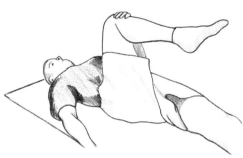

Gluteal Stretch

Lie on your back and bend your right knee to a 90-degree angle. Grab that knee with your left hand and move it across your body toward the left shoulder. The left leg stays extended, moves toward the midline of the body, and rotates internally. Exhale on the stretch phase and hold for two seconds, then return to the starting position. Repeat eight to ten times. Then, perform the same stretch with the left knee.

Double-Leg Pelvic Tilt

Lie on your back and flex your knees one at a time (avoid lifting both knees toward your chest at the same time). Grasp your legs under the knees, contract your stomach muscles, and gently pull your legs toward your chest. Exhale on the stretch phase and hold for two seconds, then return to the starting position. Repeat eight to ten times.

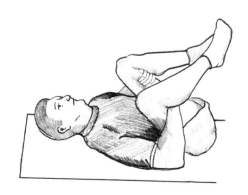

Hamstring Stretch (Bent Knee)

Lie on your back with both knees bent and feet resting flat on the floor. Lift your left leg, keeping the knee bent, and wrap a rope under the ball of the foot. From

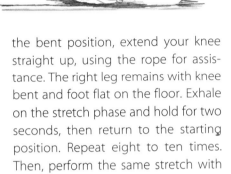

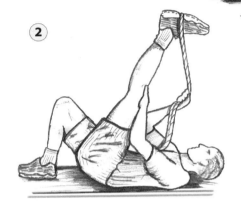

the bent position, extend your knee straight up, using the rope for assistance. The right leg remains with knee bent and foot flat on the floor. Exhale on the stretch phase and hold for two seconds, then return to the starting position. Repeat eight to ten times. Then, perform the same stretch with the right leg.

Hamstring Stretch (Straight Leg)

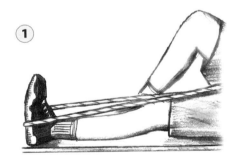

Lie on your back. Your right leg is bent with the foot flat on the floor; your left leg is straight with a rope wrapped around the ball of the foot. Contract

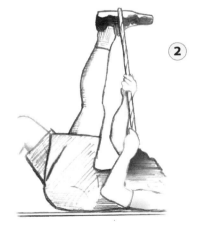

the quadriceps muscle (front of thigh) of the left leg, keeping the knee extended, and lift straight up toward the ceiling. Use the rope to assist the stretch, not to help lift the leg. Exhale on the stretch phase and hold for two seconds, then return to the starting position. Repeat eight to ten times. Then, perform the same stretch with the right leg.

Groin Stretch

Lie on your back with legs extended, and wrap a rope under the ball of your right foot and toward the inside of the ankle. The uninvolved (left) leg should be moved slightly away from the body. Using the hip muscles, move the right leg away from the middle of the body, using the rope for assistance. Keep your toes pointed toward the ceiling as the leg slides along the floor. Avoid lifting

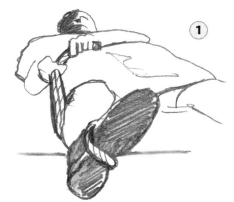

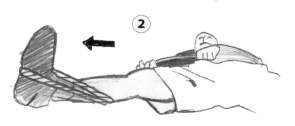

the leg during the stretch. Exhale on the stretch phase and hold for two seconds, then return to the starting position. Repeat eight to ten times. Then, perform the same stretch with the left leg.

Iliotibial Band/Hip Abductor Stretch I

Lie on your back and wrap a rope under the ball of your left foot and to the outside of the ankle. Keep both legs extended and rotate the right leg slightly inward and toward the midline

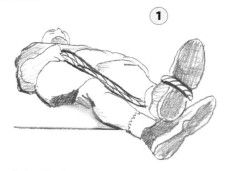

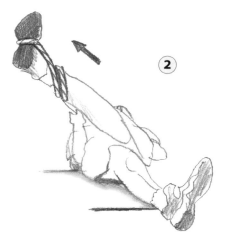

of the body. Rotate the left leg slightly outward, with the toes pointed outward. Keeping the knee extended and using the rope for assistance, move the left leg across the body to the right. Exhale on the stretch phase and hold for two seconds, then return to the starting position. Repeat eight to ten times. Then, perform the same stretch with the right leg.

Iliotibial Band/Hip Abductor Stretch II

Building on Stretch I above, this stretch involves more of the hip muscle (gluteal medius). Lie on your back and wrap the rope under the ball of your right foot and to the inside of the ankle. Keep both legs straight with your left leg turned slightly inward and moved toward

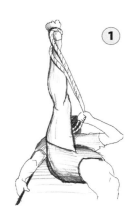

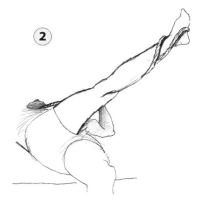

the midline of the body. Lift the right leg up until you have reached a 90-degree angle at the hip, then move

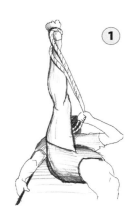

the leg directly across the body (toward the left). Keep your knee extended. Exhale on the stretch phase and hold for two seconds, then return to the starting position. Repeat eight to ten times. Then, perform the same stretch with the left leg.

Seated Low-Back Stretch

Sit with your knees shoulder-width apart and toes pointed straight ahead. Tuck your chin in and contract your abdominal muscles, then slowly bend forward toward the floor. Do not bounce at the end of the movement. Exhale on the stretch phase and hold for two seconds, then return to the starting position. Repeat eight to ten times.

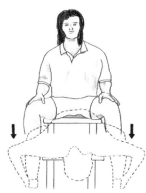

Trunk Rotation

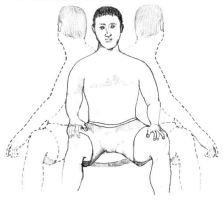

While seated, keep your hips pointed forward and gently rotate your torso to the right. Reach your right hand behind you, while the left hand assists with the rotation by gently pressing against your right leg. Exhale on the stretch phase and hold for two seconds, then return to the starting position. Repeat ten times. Then, perform the same stretch on the left side.

Exercises for the Low Back

The following exercises will help you condition your low-back muscles and recover from injury.

Straight-Leg Raise

Lie on your back with the left leg bent and relaxed. With the right leg extended, lift the leg slowly, keeping the foot flexed and toes pointed toward your chest. Exhale on the work phase, then slowly return to the starting position. Repeat ten times. Then, perform the same exercise with the left leg. You can add an ankle weight for more resistance as needed.

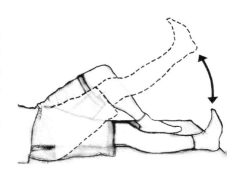

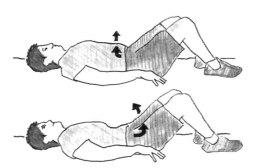

Pelvic Tilt

Lie on your back with both legs flexed and feet flat on the floor. Tilt your pelvis up and back while contracting the lower abdominal muscles. Your pelvis should be lifted slightly at the end of the movement. Exhale on the work phase and hold for three to five seconds, then return to the starting position. Repeat ten times. Place small weights on the abdomen for resistance as needed.

Pelvic Lift

Lie on your back with both knees flexed and feet flat on the floor. Contract the gluteal and low-back

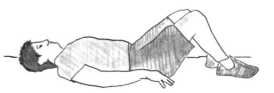

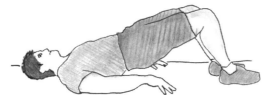

muscles and lift your pelvis. Exhale on the work phase and hold for three to five seconds, then return to the starting position. Repeat five to ten times.

Hamstring Exercise (Straight Leg)

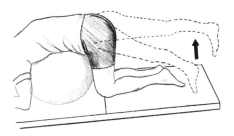

Kneel and lie forward over an exercise ball. Extend one leg back and slowly lift it toward the ceiling. Exhale on the work phase, then slowly return to the starting position. Repeat fifteen times. Add ankle weights as necessary. Then, perform the same exercise on the other leg.

Side Leg Raise for the Hips

Lie on your side with both legs extended. Lift the top leg toward the ceiling with the knee extended and foot flexed (toes pointed toward the chest). Rotate the leg slightly inward so that the heel is higher than the toes. The resting leg can be straight or slightly bent. Exhale on the work phase, then slowly return to the starting position. Repeat ten times. Then, perform the same exercise with the other leg. Add an ankle weight for more resistance as needed.

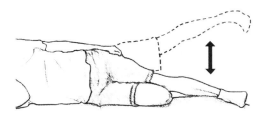

Groin (Adductor) Strengthening Exercise

Lie on your side on the floor. The left leg is extended and resting on the seat of a chair (or a bench). The right leg is underneath the chair, with knee extended and toes flexed toward the chest. Lift the right leg toward the chair, being sure to

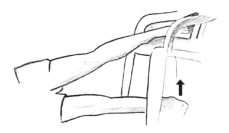

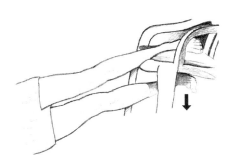

keep the toes flexed. Keep your stomach muscles slightly tightened. Exhale on the work phase, then slowly return to the starting position. Repeat ten times. Then, perform the same exercise with the left leg. Add an ankle weight for more resistance as needed.

Half Superman

Lie on your stomach on a table or mat. Lift your left arm and right leg simultaneously, then switch to lifting your right arm and left leg. As your strength improves, you can add weights to the wrists and ankles (ankle weights are best). Start with five repetitions and increase as you get stronger. Movements should be very slow and controlled; exhale on the work phase.

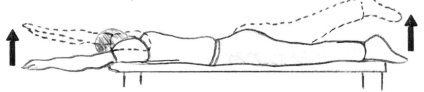

Abdominal Crunches

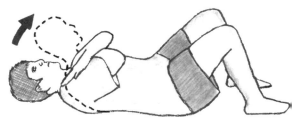

Lie on your back with your knees bent and cross your arms over your chest. Slowly lift your upper body, aiming your chin toward your belly button. Keep your pelvis tilted back toward the floor and exhale as you do the exercise. (If your abdominal muscles are too weak at first, grip under your thighs to assist lifting your upper body.) Return to the starting position and repeat fifteen times.

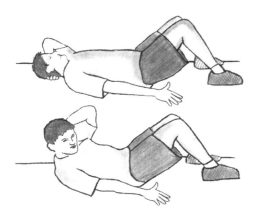

Oblique Abdominal Muscles

Lie on your back with your knees bent and place one hand behind your head. Lift up and move your head toward the opposite knee. Return to the starting position and repeat ten times. Then, perform the same exercise on the other side.

Massage Techniques for the Low Back

These massage techniques can relieve muscle spasm and pain, increase circulation, and promote the healing of low-back injuries.

Assisted Gliding Massage for the Low Back

Lie on your stomach. The massage assistant uses the palms of both hands to glide down the lower back toward the buttocks. He or she should keep the palms on the muscles on either side of the spine (not directly applying pressure to the spine).

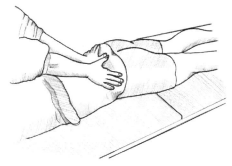

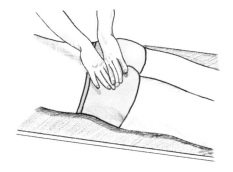

Assisted Gluteal Massage

Lie on your stomach. The massage assistant uses the fingers of both hands to gently glide down the buttock on one side. He or she starts at the edge of the sacral bone and glides downward. Repeat as necessary.

When to Call the Doctor

- If you have persistent pain or swelling
- If you experience increasing weakness
- If there is loss of bladder and bowel functions
- If you feel numbness, tingling, or coldness in your legs

Questions and Answers

Q: *Why does stretching the hamstrings help the lower back?*

A: Anatomically, the hamstrings attach underneath the gluteal (buttocks) muscles at the ischial tuberosity of the pelvic bone. As hamstring muscles tighten, they put stress on the lower back. As they continue to pull, they become weaker. Keeping the hamstrings flexible takes the tension and pressure off the bottom of the pelvis, which in turn lessens pressure and pulling on the low back. Sitting all day can cause the hamstrings to shorten or tighten due to being in a flexed position. Pressure on the spine is increased eight times while sitting as opposed to standing. For these reasons, stretching the hamstrings will help relieve back pain.

Q: *With back pain, is there a proper way to sleep and get out of bed?*

A: From an anatomical perspective, the correct way to sleep is lying on your back with a small pillow underneath the knees and a small cervical pillow or a rolled towel underneath your neck. This can be difficult for some people to do.

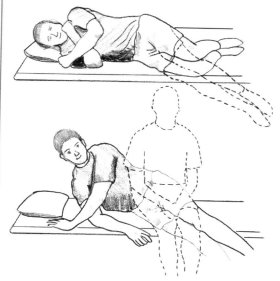

We suggest that if you sleep on your side or stomach, be willing to change your habits. If through the night you turn on your side, place the pillow between your knees. When arising in the morning, it's important to roll to your side first (facing the edge of the bed). Once on your side, slide your legs off the bed and use the top arm to push down on the mattress, lifting your upper body to a sitting position. This is the correct way to sit up from bed without worsening any pain.

FIGURE 7.4. PAIN-FREE WAY TO GET OUT OF BED

Q: *Why is it important to work my abdominal muscles? My doctor and physical therapist have told me to strengthen these muscles.*

A: Abdominal strengthening helps counterbalance the back muscles, thus distributing the stress of the back more evenly and even eliminating back pain. However, it is possible to be too strong in the front and weak in the back. Once again, it's important to create a balance.

Prevention Is the Key

• Stretch daily to stay flexible and strong.

• Avoid sitting for extended periods of time: get up and move frequently.

• Stay hydrated and eat a balanced diet to feed your muscles and body.

• Practice and learn proper lifting techniques. Avoid lifting objects that may be too heavy or wear proper safety equipment.

• Maintain your back health by routine visits to a chiropractor or massage therapist.

Chapter 8

Pain in the Upper Leg and Knee

Deirdre had been active in a variety of sports for most of her adult life. Soccer, triathlons, and rowing were important activities because they helped "recharge her batteries." In 2002, during a soccer game, she felt a "pop" in her right quadriceps muscle and the pain was immediate. Initially, she thought the injury might heal without intervention, but Deirdre eventually sought professional advice. While surgery was a consideration, she opted for nonsurgical remedies, including stretching, massage, and progressive resistance training. "Not only did these methods help the quadriceps, but I incorporated the stretching exercises into my daily athletic routine and my injury rate has decreased dramatically," says Deirdre. "And my overall flexibility and athletic performance has improved."

UPPER-LEG PAIN

Leg pain may be caused by direct trauma, overexertion, muscular imbalance, weakness, or lack of flexibility in the soft tissues (muscles, tendons, and ligaments). Conditions associated with upper-leg pain include:

- "Charley horse": contusion or bruising to the muscle belly of the quadriceps muscle

- Quadriceps strain: excessive stretch or pull to a muscle or tendon at the front of the thigh; the quadriceps is composed of four muscles—rectus femoris, vastus lateralis, vastus medialis, and vastus intermedius

- Hamstring strain or "flat tire": excessive stretch or pull to a muscle or tendon at the back of the thigh; the hamstring is comprised of three muscles—semimembranosus, semitendinosus, and biceps femoris

- Groin strain: excessive stretch or pull to the muscles on the inside of the leg; pain can gravitate toward the abdomen where it connects with the thigh

Activities such as running, football, soccer, softball, hockey, swimming, participating in a triathlon, and cycling can result in upper-leg pain, especially among so-
called weekend warriors. Leg pain is usually due to overuse or strength imbalance.
In the elderly, it is also associated with falls or trauma. Upper-leg pain may be an indication of a strained muscle, bursitis, or a chronic disease, such as cancer in the lymph
nodes (groin area) or myositis ossificans (bone formation within the quadriceps
muscle).

Stretching, exercises to strengthen the leg muscles, and massage can all help
alleviate pain in the upper leg.

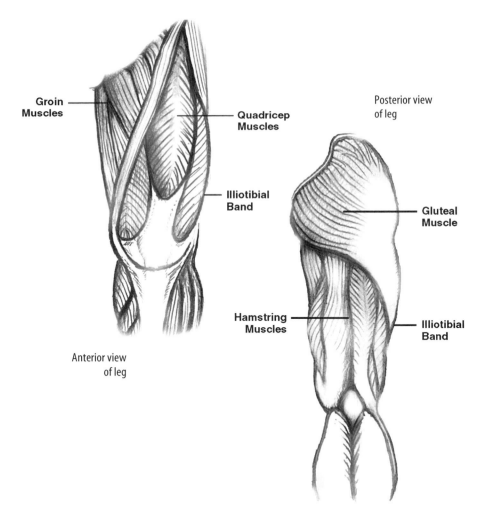

FIGURE 8.1. ANATOMY OF THE UPPER LEG

UPPER-LEG PAIN OVERVIEW	
Signs and Symptoms	**Causes**
• Bruising or discoloration	• Overexertion
• Weakness in the leg (loss of strength)	• Dehydration of the body
• Pain or tenderness	• Lack of flexibility
• Limping	• Not properly warming up before activity
• Swelling (superficial or deep) or deformity	• Muscle imbalance (one side weaker than the other)
• Muscle spasms	• Muscle weakness
	• Direct trauma

Recipe for a Healthy Upper Leg

1. Stretch one to two times daily (morning and evening usually works best); do eight to ten repetitions, holding each stretch for two seconds only. Always take your stretch back to the starting position before the next repetition; exhale your breath on the stretch phase.

2. Perform RICHES: rest, ice, compression, heat, elevation, and support (see Chapter 3).

3. Ice the affected area two to four times daily for ten minutes each time; however, be cautious of ice sensitivity. For a "charley horse," ice and stretch, using a support wrap on the injured area, if needed. Use heat (moist heat is preferred) after seventy-two hours if there's no swelling.

4. Use strengthening exercises to create a muscular balance. Exercises should be done three times weekly, with one day of rest in between. Always stretch before you strengthen.

5. Self-massage—in this case, "milking" of muscle tissue or gliding—can be applied one to two times daily; however, do not deeply massage or heat an injury within the first seventy-two hours or if swelling is present, as this can cause complications.

6. When returning to exercise, apply ice prior to exercise, followed by light stretching and a proper warm-up. You can gradually intensify the workload as the pain decreases and range of motion increases. Be sure to cool down properly, followed by light stretching and icing.

7. Maintain a proper diet and hydration for recovery (see Chapter 2).

Stretches for the Upper Leg

A number of stretches have proven effective in promoting flexibility and alleviating upper-leg pain.

Hip Flexor

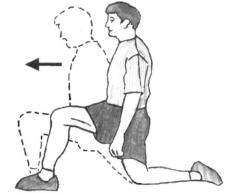

Kneel with your right knee on the floor (place a pad under the knee). Your left leg is bent at the knee with your foot flat on the ground about twelve inches in front of the left knee. Lean forward onto the flexed (left) knee until the knee is directly above your left ankle. Contract your stomach muscles as you do this movement. Exhale on the stretch phase and hold for two seconds, then return to the starting position. Repeat eight to ten times. Then, perform the same stretch with the left knee on the floor and the right knee extended.

Quadriceps Stretch

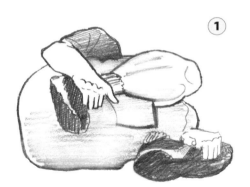

Lying on your left side, bend your bottom (left) leg and reach the knee toward your chest. Grasp under your foot with your left hand, if possible. Bend your top (right) leg and grab the ankle with your right hand. Contract the gluteus muscles (buttocks) and stomach muscles, then reach the top (right) leg backward as far as you can. It is important to keep your leg parallel to the floor as you stretch the leg backwards. Exhale on the stretch phase and hold for two seconds, then return to the starting position. Repeat eight to ten times. Then, perform the same stretch on the left leg (while lying on your right side).

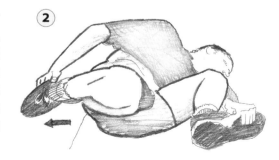

Hamstring Stretch (Bent Knee)

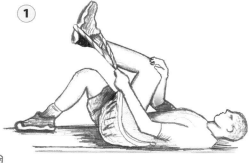

Lie on your back with both knees bent and feet resting flat on the floor. Lift your left leg, keeping the knee bent, and wrap a rope under the ball of the foot. From

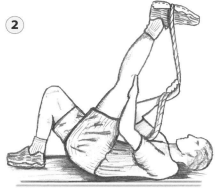

the bent position, extend your knee straight up, using the rope for gentle assistance. The right leg remains with knee bent and foot flat on the floor. Exhale on the stretch phase and hold for two seconds, then return to the starting position. Repeat eight to ten times. Then, perform the same stretch with the right leg.

Hamstring Stretch (Straight Leg)

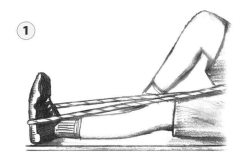

Lie on your back. Your right leg is bent with the foot flat on the floor; your left leg is straight with a rope wrapped around the ball of the foot. Contract

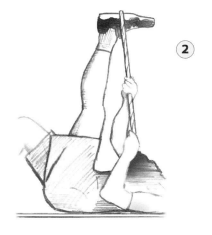

the quadriceps muscle (front of thigh) of the left leg, keeping the knee extended, and lift straight up toward the ceiling. Use the rope to assist the stretch, not to help lift the leg. Exhale on the stretch phase and hold for two seconds, then return to the starting position. Repeat eight to ten times. Then, perform the same stretch with the right leg.

Groin Stretch

Lie on your back with legs extended, and wrap a rope under the ball of your right foot and toward the inside of the ankle. The uninvolved (left) leg should be moved slightly away from the body. Using the hip muscles, move the right leg away from the middle of the body, using the rope for assistance. Keep your toes pointed toward the ceiling as the leg slides along the floor. Avoid lifting

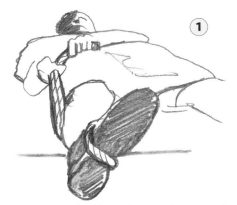

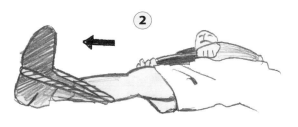

the leg during the stretch. Exhale on the stretch phase and hold for two seconds, then return to the starting position. Repeat eight to ten times. Then, perform the same stretch with the left leg.

Iliotibial Band/Hip Abductor Stretch I

Lie on your back and wrap a rope under the ball of your left foot and to the outside of the ankle. Keep both legs extended and rotate the right leg slightly inward and toward the midline

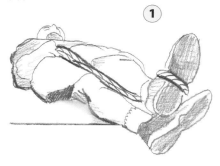

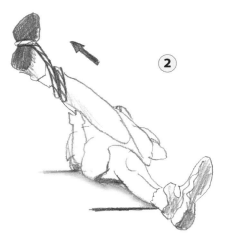

of the body. Rotate the left leg slightly outward, with the toes pointed outward. Keeping the knee extended and using the rope for assistance, move the left leg across the body to the right. Exhale on the stretch phase and hold for two seconds, then return to the starting position. Repeat eight to ten times. Then, perform the same stretch with the right leg.

Iliotibial Band/Hip Abductor Stretch II

Building on Stretch I above, this stretch involves more of the hip muscle (gluteal medius). Lie on your back and wrap the rope under the ball of your right foot and to the inside of the ankle. Keep both legs straight with your left leg turned slightly inward and moved toward

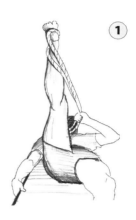

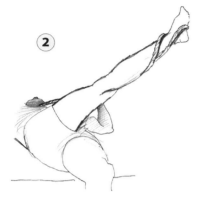

the midline of the body. Lift the right leg up until you have reached a 90-degree angle at the hip, then move the leg directly across the body (toward the left). Keep your knee extended. Exhale on the stretch phase and hold for two seconds, then return to the starting position. Repeat eight to ten times. Then, perform the same stretch with the left leg.

Gluteal Stretch

Lie on your back and bend your right knee to a 90-degree angle. Grab that knee with your left hand and move it across your body toward the left shoulder. The left leg stays extended, moves toward the midline of the body, and rotates internally. Exhale on the stretch phase and hold for

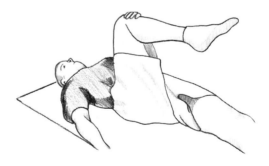

two seconds, then return to the starting position. Repeat eight to ten times. Then, perform the same stretch with the left knee.

Exercises for the Upper Leg

The following exercises will help you condition your upper-leg muscles and recover from injury.

Straight-Leg Raise

Lie on your back with the left leg bent and relaxed. With the right leg extended, lift the leg slowly keeping the foot flexed and toes pointed toward your chest. Exhale on the work phase, then slowly return to the starting position. Repeat ten times. Then, perform the same exercise with the left leg. You can add an ankle weight for more resistance as needed.

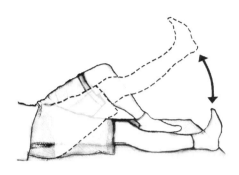

Hamstring Curls (Bent)

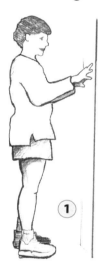

Use a table or the wall as a stabilizing support. Place the left foot on a two-inch-high block—this will allow the right leg a full range of motion. Flex the right knee to a 90-degree angle, then return to the starting position. To isolate the internal and external hamstring muscles, turn the right leg inward for a set of ten repetitions, then turn it outward for a set of ten repetitions. Then, perform the same exercise with the left leg. Add ankle weights as necessary.

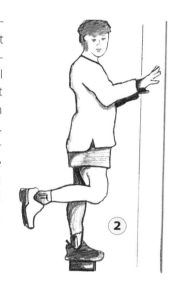

Groin (Adductor) Strengthening Exercise

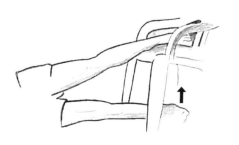

Lie on your side on the floor. The left leg is extended and resting on the seat of a chair (or a bench). The right leg is underneath the chair, with knee extended and toes flexed toward the chest. Lift the right leg toward the chair, being sure to keep the toes flexed.

Keep your stomach muscles slightly tightened. Exhale on the work phase, then slowly return to the starting position. Repeat ten times. Then, perform the same exercise with the left leg. Add an ankle weight for more resistance as needed.

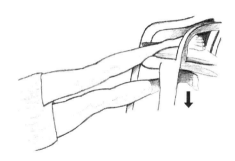

Side Leg Raise for the Hips

Lie on your side with both legs extended. Lift the top leg toward the ceiling with the knee extended and foot flexed (toes pointed toward the chest). Rotate the leg slightly inward so that the heel is higher than the toes. The resting leg can be

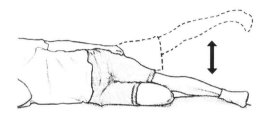

straight or slightly bent. Exhale on the work phase, then slowly return to the starting position. Repeat ten times. Then, perform the same exercise with the other leg. Add an ankle weight for more resistance as needed.

Wall Slides

Stand with your back against a wall. Move your feet slightly forward and in line with your shoulders. Bending your knees, slowly slide down the wall until your knees flex to a 90-degree angle and slowly return to the starting position. Exhale on the work phase. Repeat ten times. Hold weights in your hands for extra resistance as needed.

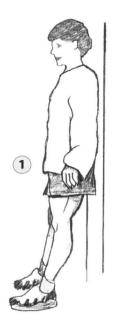

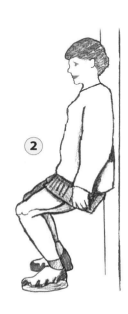

Massage Techniques for the Upper Leg

These massage techniques can relieve muscle spasm and pain, increase circulation, and promote the healing of upper-leg injuries.

Gliding Iliotibial-Band Massage

Sit with your leg extended. Stroke the leg from the thigh down toward the foot, using long, circular movements. Repeat as necessary.

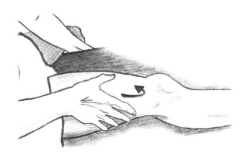

Assisted Gliding Iliotibial-Band Massage

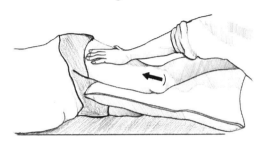

Lie on your side with a pillow between your knees. The massage assistant will use the palm of his or her hand to gently glide along the iliotibial band, starting at the knee and working up the thigh. Exhale during the gliding phase. Repeat as necessary.

Flushing of Hamstrings (Assisted Massage)

Lie on your stomach. The massage assistant gently holds your left ankle in one hand, keeping the knee slightly flexed. His or her other hand is placed just above

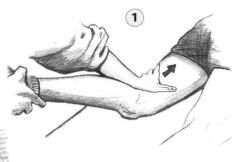

the knee (direct pressure should not be placed on the back of the knee). He or she glides the hand forward up the thigh while simultaneously lowering the leg. Repeat as necessary on both legs.

Flushing of Quadriceps Muscle (Assisted Massage)

Lie on your back. The massage assistant uses both hands to glide along the quadriceps muscle (front of the thigh). The gliding stroke should start just above the knee and move toward the top of the quadriceps muscle. Repeat as necessary on both legs.

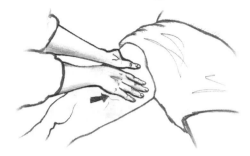

When to Call the Doctor

• If you have persistent pain

• If you experience numbness or tingling, especially down the side of the leg

• If there is loss of function or decreased range of motion

• When you have loss of circulation (cold feet or no pulse)

Questions and Answers

Q: *How soon can I get back to activity with a pulled hamstring muscle?*

A: It's important to be able to classify the severity of the pull before the assessment can be made.

Mild—slightly pulled muscle; no tearing or apparent loss of muscle strength

Moderate—some tearing of the muscle fibers or the tendon; no apparent loss of strength

Severe—the muscle or tendon has been completely torn or ruptured at the attachment

Typically, for mild and sometimes moderate strains, activity can be resumed in two to four weeks, gradually, as long as the following criteria are met: bilateral (both sides of the body) strength, increased range of motion (flexibility), and little to no pain during or after activity. Make sure to warm up properly before exercise and cool down after exercise. Consult with your athletic trainer or physical therapist for a follow-up visit if necessary.

Q: *What can I do to prevent a groin pull?*

A: The best way to prevent any muscle pull is to maintain proper flexibility (overall) and strength. The adductor muscles (commonly known as the groin muscles) assist the hamstring muscles when they are fatigued or injured. If you exercise regularly to muscle fatigue without proper cool down or days of rest, the muscles are left with fatigue and sometimes become strained or weak. When a muscle "gives up," other muscles participate in the activity to help achieve a balance. If a muscle is not strong enough to perform the substituted action, it will pull or become strained. Some individuals achieve flexibility a little easier than others, due to genetics and overall health. Keep in mind, however, that even those who are extremely flexible still must work on their strength and muscle balance.

Prevention Is the Key

- Warm up before you exercise: remember to stretch first, both the front and back of the legs; always maintain a balance.

- Use correct exercise technique or form.

- Don't overlook injury or a minor pain or twinge: avoidance can lead to lifetime complications (for example, arthritis).

- Proper footwear is critical for any sport or activity.

KNEE PAIN

Rose exercised regularly for ten years. Then, at age fifty-three, she decided to start jogging. In the beginning she found it easy, but after four months she developed pain in the iliotibial band and "clicking" in her knees. Massage helped in the short-term, but the clicking in her knees would quickly return. Rose came to see me (Kim) and I told her, "I'm not going to fix your knees—you are going to do this yourself, and I'll show you how." I worked on her legs and taught her a stretching routine to increase her flexibility and to help stabilize her knees.

"After using the stretching routine for one week, the pain in my leg had eased and walking was much more comfortable," says Rose. Within three weeks, she could run with only minor pain; after five weeks, her knees were stable and running was painless. "Since then, I have used stretching routines to deal with other leg-muscle flare-ups from running. These routines are essential to my ability to remain active without injury."

Knee pain may be the result of direct trauma, overuse, or other contributing factors such as violent movement, poor exercise surface, or incorrect biomechanics (body movement). Conditions associated with knee pain include:

- Water on the knee: inflammation of the bursa in the knee (Bursas are located in front of the kneecap, on both sides of the knee below the joint line, and behind the patellar and hamstring tendons.)

- Runner's knee/jumper's knee: tendinitis below the kneecap located in the patellar tendon

- Kneecap (patella) irritation: pain beneath the kneecap; can cause discomfort while bending or going down stairs

- Lateral knee pain: tightness in the iliotibial (IT) band, the thick band of tissue that originates at the hip and attaches to the outside of the knee; causes discomfort while bending the knee, running, or going down stairs

- Joint-line knee pain: damage to cartilage in the knee that causes a "locking" or catching sensation

- Deep knee pain: deep pain within and behind the knee, usually representative of a torn anterior cruciate ligament (ACL)

- Sprain to ligaments: stretch or tear to the ligaments of the knee; pain is usually located on the inside or outside of the knee joint

- Osgood-Schlatter's disease: tenderness, pain, or swelling below the kneecap at the little bony structure called the tibia tubercle (the tubercle can appear swollen and warm); most commonly seen in adolescents

Knee pain is most prevalent in sports involving running or jumping, such as football; it is also common in cycling and hiking. There were approximately 650,000 knee injuries treated in United States hospitals in 2001. Knee pain usually indicates soft-tissue injury to ligaments or tendons. Direct trauma and twisting motions lead to most ligamentous injuries, but in older patients, cysts can sometimes form in the posterior (back) side of the knee and rupture the popliteal tendon (the tendon behind the knee joint).

Stretching, exercises to strengthen the muscles around the knee, and massage can all help alleviate knee pain.

Recipe for a Healthy Knee

1. Stretch up to three times daily, focusing on the gluteals (buttocks), hamstrings, quadriceps, IT band (hip abductor), and hip adductors; hold each stretch for no more than two seconds and repeat eight to ten times. Always take your stretch back to the starting position before the next repetition; exhale your breath on the stretch phase.

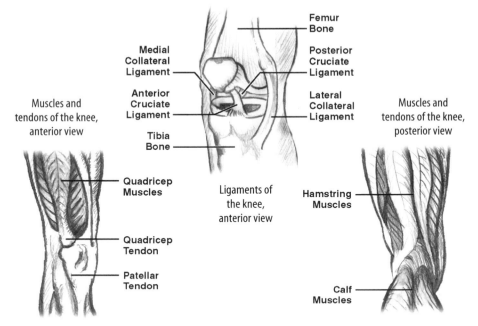

FIGURE 8.2. ANATOMY OF THE KNEE

KNEE PAIN OVERVIEW

Signs and Symptoms

- Pain and tenderness before or after activity
- Trouble walking
- Instability or weakness in joint
- A "popping" sound in the knee
- Catching or locking of the knee
- Point tenderness
- Swelling of the knee joint
- Deformity

Causes

- Direct trauma
- Overuse, especially knee extension or jumping
- Twisting motion
- Excessive kneeling
- Excessive weight bearing from obesity
- Genetics
- Poor posture or biomechanics (body movement)
- A condition such as bowleg, knock-knee, or hyperextended knee
- Osgood-Schlatter's disease

2. Perform RICHES: rest, ice, compression, heat, elevation, and support (see Chapter 3).

3. Do strengthening exercises (especially hamstrings) three times a week, with one day of rest in between. Always stretch before you strengthen.

4. Ice massage or apply an ice bag on the knee joint two to four times daily for ten minutes; be aware of ice sensitivity. An Ace wrap or knee sleeve can provide additional support, if needed.

5. Massage techniques, particularly "milking" of the quadriceps muscles and applying friction around the patella, can be applied one to two times daily.

6. When returning to exercise, apply ice prior to exercise, followed by light stretching and a proper warm-up. You can gradually intensify the workload as the pain decreases and range of motion increases. Be sure to cool down properly, followed by light stretching and icing.

7. Be aware of playing surfaces: cement, asphalt, artificial turf, rubber, or cushion. Soft ground is usually the best surface for running.

8. Wear supportive shoes with the appropriate shoe insert; see a podiatrist or biomechanics specialist for a "casted" shoe insert.

9. Maintain a proper diet and hydration for recovery (see Chapter 2).

Stretches for the Knee

A number of stretches have proven effective in promoting flexibility and alleviating knee pain.

Gluteal Stretch

Lie on your back and bend your right knee to a 90-degree angle. Grab that knee with your left hand and move it across your body toward the left shoulder. The left leg stays extended, moves toward the midline of 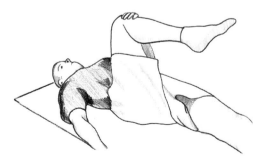 the body, and rotates internally. Exhale on the stretch phase and hold for two seconds, then return to the starting position. Repeat eight to ten times. Then, perform the same stretch with the left knee.

Calf Stretch

Place a rope around the ball of your right foot, and sit on the floor with your leg extended (the knee should be straight). The opposite leg should be bent to help ease any low-back or hamstring discomfort. Bring the top of your right foot toward your chest, using the rope to assist. Avoid leaning

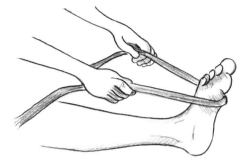

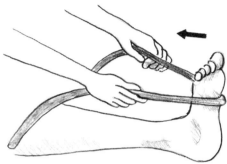

back while assisting yourself during the stretch phase. Maintain a 90-degree angle at the hip, using your arms only to assist yourself with the rope. Exhale on the stretch phase and hold for two seconds, then return to the starting position. Repeat eight to ten times. Then, repeat the stretch with the left leg.

Hamstring Stretch (Bent Knee)

Lie on your back with both knees bent and feet resting flat on the floor. Lift your left leg, keeping the knee bent, and wrap a rope under the ball of the foot. From

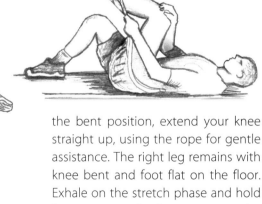

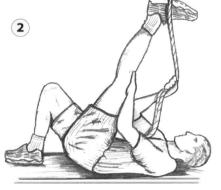

the bent position, extend your knee straight up, using the rope for gentle assistance. The right leg remains with knee bent and foot flat on the floor. Exhale on the stretch phase and hold for two seconds, then return to the starting position. Repeat eight to ten times. Then, perform the same stretch with the right leg.

Hamstring Stretch (Straight Leg)

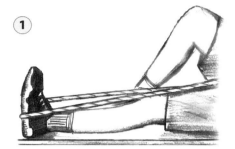

Lie on your back. Your right leg is bent with the foot flat on the floor; your left leg is straight with a rope wrapped around the ball of the foot. Contract

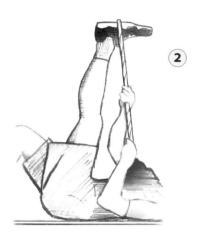

the quadriceps muscle (front of thigh) of the left leg, keeping the knee extended, and lift straight up toward the ceiling. Use the rope to assist the stretch, not to help lift the leg. Exhale on the stretch phase and hold for two seconds, then return to the starting position. Repeat eight to ten times. Then, perform the same stretch with the right leg

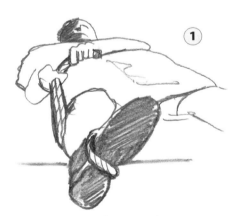

Groin Stretch

Lie on your back with legs extended, and wrap a rope under the ball of your right foot and toward the inside of the ankle. The uninvolved (left) leg should be moved slightly away from the body. Using the hip muscles, move the right leg away from the middle of the body, using the rope for assistance. Keep your toes pointed toward the ceiling as the leg slides along the floor. Avoid lifting

the leg during the stretch. Exhale on the stretch phase and hold for two seconds, then return to the starting position. Repeat eight to ten times. Then, perform the same stretch with the left leg.

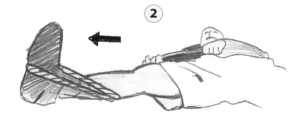

Iliotibial Band/Hip Abductor Stretch I

Lie on your back and wrap a rope under the ball of your left foot and to the outside of the ankle. Keep both legs extended and rotate the right leg slightly inward and toward the midline

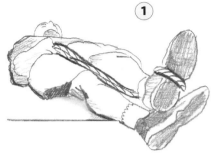

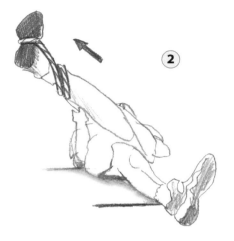

of the body. Rotate the left leg slightly outward, with the toes pointed outward. Keeping the knee extended and using the rope for assistance, move the left leg across the body to the right. Exhale on the stretch phase and hold for two seconds, then return to the starting position. Repeat eight to ten times. Then, perform the same stretch with the right leg.

Iliotibial Band/Hip Abductor Stretch II

Building on Stretch I above, this stretch involves more of the hip muscle (gluteal medius). Lie on your back and wrap the rope under the ball of your right foot and to the inside of the ankle. Keep both legs straight with your left leg turned slightly inward and moved toward

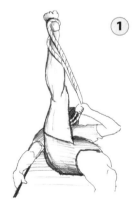

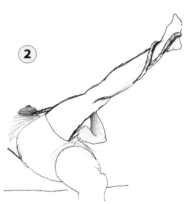

the midline of the body. Lift the right leg up until you have reached a 90-degree angle at the hip, then move the leg directly across the body (toward the left). Keep your knee extended. Exhale on the stretch phase and hold for two seconds, then return to the starting position. Repeat eight to ten times. Then, perform the same stretch with the left leg.

Hip Flexor

Kneel with your right knee on the floor (place a pad under the knee). Your left leg is bent at the knee with your foot flat on the ground about twelve inches in front of the left knee. Lean forward onto the flexed (left) knee until the knee is directly above your left ankle. Contract your stomach muscles as you do this movement. Exhale on the stretch phase and hold for two seconds, then return

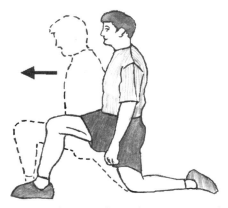

to the starting position. Repeat eight to ten times. Then, perform the same stretch with the left knee on the floor and the right knee extended.

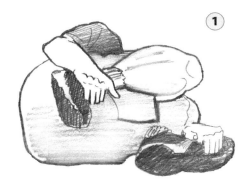

Quadriceps Stretch

Lying on your left side, bend your bottom (left) leg and reach the knee toward your chest. Grasp under your foot with your left hand, if possible. Bend your top (right) leg and grab the ankle with your right hand. Contract the gluteus muscles (buttocks) and stomach muscles, then reach the top (right) leg backward

as far as you can. It is important to keep your leg parallel to the floor as you stretch the leg backwards. Exhale on the stretch phase and hold for two seconds, then return to the starting position. Repeat eight to ten times. Then, perform the same stretch on the left leg (while lying on your right side).

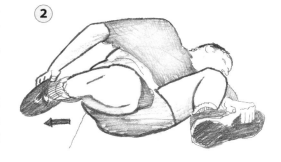

Exercises for the Knee

The following exercises will help you condition your knee muscles and recover from injury.

Straight-Leg Raise

Lie on your back with the left leg bent and relaxed. With the right leg extended, lift the leg slowly keeping the foot flexed and toes pointed toward your chest. Exhale on the work phase, then slowly return to the starting position. Repeat ten times. Then, perform the same exercise with the left leg. You can add an ankle weight for more resistance as needed.

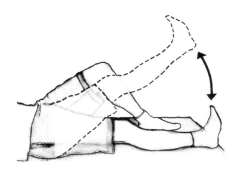

Quadriceps Exercise

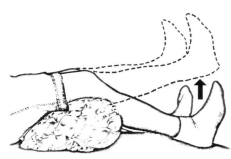

Lie on your back with a six- to eight-inch-high pillow under your knees. Begin with the legs flexed and your heels resting on the floor. Flex both the feet and toes toward the chest and straighten the legs. Hold for three to five seconds, then relax. Repeat fifteen times. Add ankle weights as necessary.

Groin (Adductor) Strengthening Exercise

Lie on your side on the floor. The left leg is extended and resting on the seat of a chair (or a bench). The right leg is underneath the chair, with knee extended and toes flexed toward the chest. Lift the right leg toward the chair, being sure to

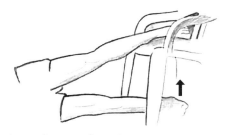

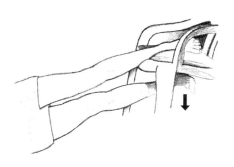

keep the toes flexed. Keep your stomach muscles slightly tightened. Exhale on the work phase, then slowly return to the starting position. Repeat ten times. Then, perform the same exercise with the left leg. Add an ankle weight for more resistance as needed.

Side Leg Raise for the Hips

Lie on your side with both legs extended. Lift the top leg toward the ceiling with the knee extended and foot flexed (toes pointed toward the chest). Rotate the leg slightly inward so that the heel is higher than the 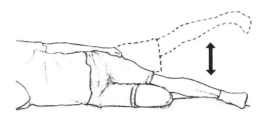 toes. The resting leg can be straight or slightly bent. Exhale on the work phase, then slowly return to the starting position. Repeat ten times. Then perform the same exercise with the other leg. Add an ankle weight for more resistance as needed.

Hamstring Curls (Bent)

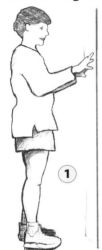

Use a table or the wall as a stabilizing support. Place the left foot on a two-inch-high block—this will allow the right leg a full range of motion. Flex the right knee to a 90-degree angle, then return to the starting position. To isolate the internal and external hamstring muscles, turn the right leg inward for a set of ten repetitions, then turn it outward for a set of ten repetitions. Then, perform the same exercise with the left leg. Add ankle weights as necessary.

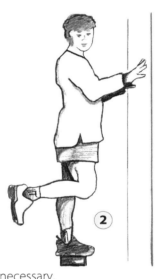

Calf Raises

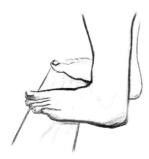

Place the ball of the foot and the toes on a two-inch-high board. Heels should rest on the floor. Hold on to the wall or a chair for support and raise up onto your toes. To isolate the inner and outer calf muscles, turn your toes inward and raise up for ten repetitions, then turn your toes outward and raise up for ten repetitions. Exhale on the work phase.

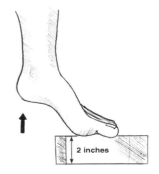

2 inches

Pelvic Lift

Lie on your back with both knees flexed. Contract the gluteal and low-back muscles and lift your pelvis. Exhale on the work phase

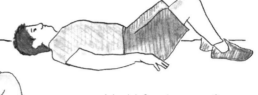

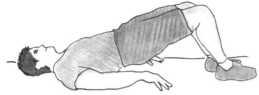

and hold for three to five seconds, then return to the starting position. Repeat five to ten times.

Massage Techniques for the Knee

These massage techniques can relieve muscle spasm and pain, increase circulation, and promote the healing of knee injuries.

Friction to Knee Joint

Place both thumbs firmly down on the tendon just above the knee and move your thumbs in a side-to-side motion. Repeat as necessary.

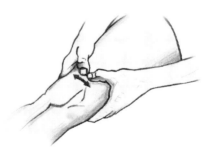

Flushing of Quadriceps Muscle (Assisted Massage)

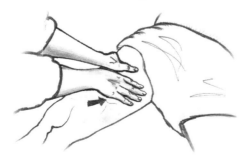

Lie on your back. The massage assistant uses both hands to glide along the quadriceps muscle (front of the thigh). The gliding stroke should start just above the knee and move toward the top of the quadriceps muscle. Repeat as necessary on both legs.

When to Call the Doctor

- If you have severe pain behind the knee or persistent pain before, during, or after exercise

- If you experience loss of function or the knee continues to "give way"

- If there is continued swelling or redness

Questions and Answers

Q: *Why do doctors order MRIs for knee injuries?*

A: MRI stands for "magnetic resonance imaging," which provides physicians with images that show damage to the bones and soft tissues, such as muscles, tendons, cartilage, ligaments, and nerves. X-rays only show the structure of bones, not soft tissues or nerves. The MRI is a noninvasive procedure and usually takes about forty-five minutes to one hour.

Q: *What is a "blown-out" knee and how long does it take to recover?*

A: A "blown-out" knee usually indicates a torn anterior cruciate ligament (ACL), which connects the femur (thigh bone) and tibia (shin bone) and torn medial collateral ligament and medial meniscus (cartilage). The ACL is found deep within the knee joint—most patients will indicate that they heard or felt a "pop" during the injury. Injury mechanisms include twisting with a blow and direct trauma to the outside of the knee. ACL tears are occurring in epidemic proportions among female athletes, which is attributed to poor balance of quadriceps and hamstring strength, poor landing mechanisms, or the angle of knees or hips. It also has been theorized that lack of flexibility to hamstring muscles at the insertion (behind the knee joint) does not allow proper rotation of the knee. Maintaining proper flexibility and strength can often prevent injury and protect the joint during athletic activities. ACL injuries require surgical repair and rehabilitation ranging from six to nine months up to one year or more. The key to recovery is to regain full extension as soon as possible.

Q: *What are knee braces for and where can I find them?*

A: Braces support soft tissues, such as muscles, tendons, and ligaments. Some braces are made to protect against injury (such as those commonly worn by football players). Knee braces can be ordered by mail, from your doctor, or found in some sporting goods stores. The patellar tendon strap or Cho-Pat strap relieves the pressure on the patellar tendon just below the kneecap. Typical knee sleeves give support, prevent swelling, and help keep the knee joint warm. Consult with your physician, athletic trainer, or physical therapist for a proper sleeve and fitting.

Prevention Is the Key

• Always warm up before exercise or sporting activities: remember to stretch both the front and back of the legs, calves, low back, hips, and feet.

• Use correct exercise technique and form.

• Make sure you have the proper equipment for your sport, particularly shoes and shoe inserts. Also, check the treads on your shoes to make sure they are not worn through.

• Do not overlook an injury or avoid symptoms: react immediately to start the healing process and avoid any possible complications.

Chapter 9

Pain in the Lower Leg, Ankle, and Foot

Tony had competed in track and field at the highest level for six years when he tore his Achilles tendon (he had a 50 percent tear) while training for the 2000 Olympic Games. He flew back from Japan and came to see me (Kim). He started his rehabilitation immediately with regular massage and acupuncture treatments. In the following weeks, I worked with Tony to improve flexibility in the calf and lower-leg area as well as to realign the fibers in the tendon itself. The rehabilitation was a long one, but Tony was able to compete at the next Olympics in Sydney, Australia.

LOWER-LEG PAIN

Lower-leg pain may be the result of direct trauma, a complete or incomplete break of the tibia (shin bone), overstretching, or overexertion of the muscles or tendons. Conditions associated with lower-leg pain include:

- Calf strain: strain or injury to the muscles or tendons in the back of the lower leg

- Calf "cramping": muscle spasm in the back of the lower leg causing severe pain and discomfort; occurs commonly in the evenings but may occur anytime

- Shin splints: pain in front of the shin that radiates up and down the bone; may cause a stress fracture to the bone, if very severe

- Achilles tendinitis: inflammation of the Achilles tendon, which attaches the lower-leg muscles to the heel

Lower-leg pain may be caused by sports that involve running or contact, such as gymnastics, martial arts, track-and-field sports, running or jogging, cycling, and basketball. Lower-leg pain can also indicate certain health conditions, such as deep vein thrombosis, diabetes, poor circulation, and neurological deficits. It is estimated that there were over 450,000 cases of lower-leg injuries in the United States in 2001. There is a higher incidence of lower-leg injuries among younger and middle-aged people, probably due to increased activity levels.

Stretching, exercises to strengthen the lower-leg muscles, and massage can all help alleviate pain in the lower leg.

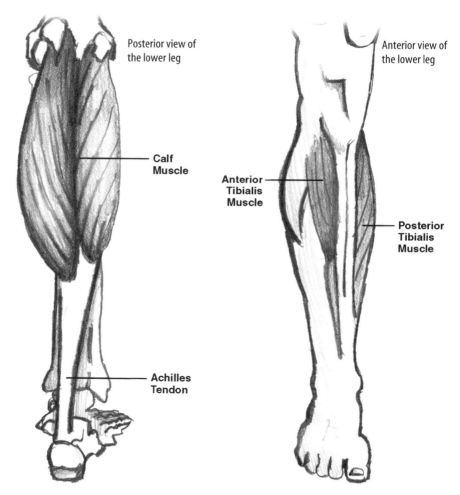

FIGURE 9.1. ANATOMY OF THE LOWER LEG

Recipe for a Healthy Lower Leg

1. Start each day by stretching your lower-leg muscles (especially before and after activity) to get them warmed up and flexible; hold each stretch for two seconds

LOWER-LEG PAIN OVERVIEW

Signs and Symptoms

- Tenderness, swelling, or heat
- Pain while in motion or still
- A "popping" sound in the muscle or tendon
- Limping
- Loss of arch on the bottom of the foot
- Muscle spasms
- Pain in the front of the leg, or along the back or inner side of the shin

Causes

- Overuse or overexertion of the muscle
- Dehydration or an imbalance of electrolytes or minerals
- Inflammation of muscles or tendons, usually due to an imbalance of the calf muscles
- Weakness or loss of strength
- Not properly warming up before activity
- Inflexibility of muscles
- Improper biomechanics (body movement)

only, and repeat eight to ten times. Always return to the starting position before the next repetition and exhale your breath on the stretch phase.

2. Strengthening exercises for the leg can be done two to three times weekly, with one day of rest in between. Always stretch before you strengthen.

3. Massage with ice or apply ice bags or packs two to four times daily for ten minutes each time (especially after exercise).

4. Massage therapy can be used one to two times daily; for severe strains, avoid deep massage techniques during the first seventy-two hours after injury.

5. Make sure that your shoes and equipment fit properly for your activity or sport. Good supportive shoes are critical for preventing leg pain.

6. When returning to exercise or activity, stretch and warm up first. Exercise or engage in sporting activities on good surfaces to prevent leg problems. Gradually increase your exercise level as symptoms and pain begin to dissipate. Always cool down properly, stretching and applying ice when finished.

7. Maintain a proper diet and hydration for recovery (see Chapter 2). Also, be sure to stay hydrated and keep your electrolytes balanced when engaged in sports or other activities.

Stretches for the Lower Leg

A number of stretches have proven effective in promoting flexibility and alleviating lower-leg pain.

Calf Stretch

Place a rope around the ball of your right foot, and sit on the floor with your leg extended (the knee should be straight). The opposite leg should be bent to help ease any low-back or hamstring discomfort. Bring the top of your right foot toward your chest, using the rope to assist. Avoid leaning

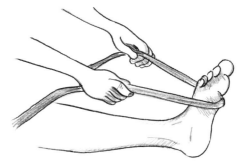

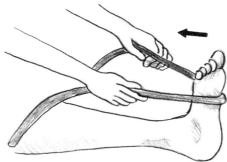

back while assisting yourself during the stretch phase. Maintain a 90-degree angle at the hip, using your arms only to assist yourself with the rope. Exhale on the stretch phase and hold for two seconds, then return to the starting position. Repeat eight to ten times. Then, repeat the stretch with the left leg.

Soleus Stretch

Sit on the floor with your knee flexed and your foot resting on the floor. Lift the foot toward your chest while keeping the heel on the floor. Assist the

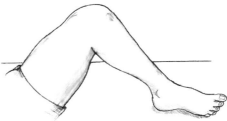

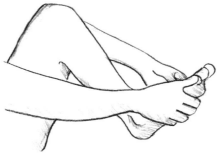

stretch with your hands under the ball of the foot (may use a rope, if necessary). Exhale on the stretch phase and hold for two seconds, then return to the starting position. Repeat eight to ten times. Then, perform the stretch with the other foot.

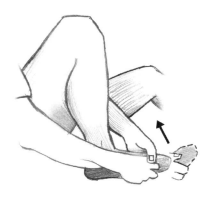

Achilles Tendon Stretch

Sit on the floor and flex one knee, bringing your heel as close as possible to your buttocks. Flex your forefoot and toes toward your chest, assisting with your hands under the ball of the foot (may use a rope, if necessary). Exhale on the stretch phase and hold for two seconds, then return to the starting position. Repeat eight to ten times. Then, perform the stretch with the other foot.

Extension of Toes

While seated, flex one knee and gently bring your heel toward your buttocks. Extend each toe back as far as possible, assisting with your hand. Exhale on the stretch phase and hold for two seconds, then return to the starting position. Repeat eight to ten times. Then, perform the stretch with the other foot. (Extending the toes also stretches the arch of the foot.)

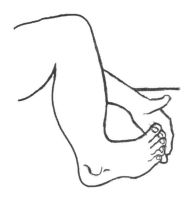

Plantar Flexion Stretch

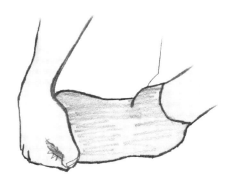

While seated, flex the left knee and place the ankle across the knee of the opposite leg. Place your right hand on top of the foot and point the foot, gently assisting with your hand. This will stretch the shin

muscle. Exhale on the stretch phase and hold for two seconds, then return to the starting position. Repeat eight to ten times. Then, perform the same stretch with the right leg.

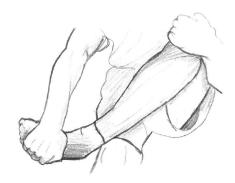

Ankle Inversion and Eversion Stretch

While seated, wrap a rope around the ball of your foot. Turn the ankle inward and flex your toes and foot toward your chest, gently assisting with the rope. Exhale on the stretch phase and hold for two seconds, then return to the

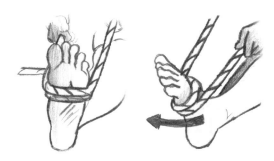

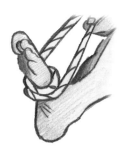

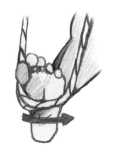

starting position. Repeat eight to ten times. Then, turn the ankle outward, again flexing the foot and gently assisting the stretch with the rope. Exhale on the stretch phase and hold for two seconds, then return to the starting position. Repeat eight to ten times. Perform the same stretch on the other foot.

Exercises for the Lower Leg

The following exercises will help you condition your lower-leg muscles and recover from injury.

Calf Raises

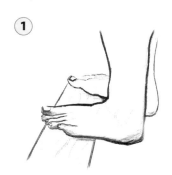

Place the ball of the foot and the toes on a two-inch-high board. Heels should rest on the floor. Hold on to the wall or a chair for support and raise up onto your toes. To isolate the inner and outer calf muscles, turn your toes inward and raise up for ten repetitions, then turn your toes outward and raise up for ten repetitions. Exhale on the work phase.

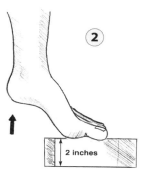

2 inches

Toe Scrunches

Place a towel on the floor with a small weight placed on top at one end of the towel. Grasp the towel with your toes, pulling the weight toward your heel. You may need to dampen your toes for a better grip. When finished, straighten the towel and repeat ten to fifteen times. Then, perform the exercise with the other foot.

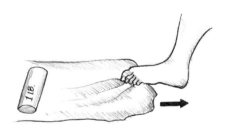

Dorsiflexion Exercise I

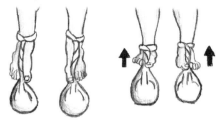

Place a small weight in a tube sock (or pillowcase) and tie the end of the sock around your ankle, feeding it between the big toe and second toe. Tie another weighted sock around your other ankle. Sit on an elevated platform, such as a tall table, so that the feet do not touch the floor and the weighted tube socks just skim the surface of the floor. Then, lift up ankles and feet. Return to the starting position and repeat fifteen times. Add more weight if necessary.

Dorsiflexion Exercise II

Follow the instructions for dorsiflexion exercise I above, with the following variation: Turn your ankles outward while lifting your ankles and feet upward. Repeat fifteen times. Add more weight if necessary.

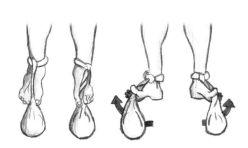

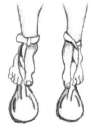
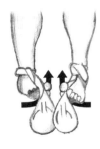

Dorsiflexion Exercise III

Follow the instructions for dorsiflexion exercise I above, with the following variation: Turn your ankles inward while lifting your ankles and feet upward. Repeat fifteen times. Add more weight if necessary.

Massage Techniques for the Lower Leg

These massage techniques can relieve muscle spasm and pain, increase circulation, and promote the healing of lower-leg injuries.

Calf Self-Massage

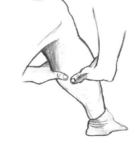

While seated with the knee flexed, glide your thumbs up the middle of the calf muscle. Start at the Achilles heel and work toward the back of the knee. Repeat as necessary.

Calf Muscle Assisted Massage

The massage assistant uses his or her thumbs to glide up the middle of the calf muscle, starting at the Achilles heel and working toward the back of the knee. Repeat as necessary.

Shin Muscle Assisted Massage

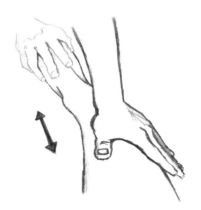

The massage assistant places one hand gently on the top of the foot. With the other hand, he or she uses the palm surface of his or her hand to massage the shin muscle (not the shin bone). The massage assistant should simultaneously glide one hand up the shin while pointing the foot and toes down with the other hand (using gentle pressure). Repeat as necessary.

When to Call the Doctor

- If you have persistent pain in spite of therapy
- If you experience numbness or tingling in the leg
- If there is any deformity or severe swelling
- If you experience loss of function or weight-bearing ability

---

Questions and Answers

Q: *What other conditions are associated with the lower leg?*

A: There are several health problems that can occur in the lower leg:

- Blood clots
- Compartment syndrome: severe swelling in the lower leg
- "Drop foot": damage to the peroneal nerve; prevents you from lifting up your foot
- Phlebitis: inflammation of the veins; commonly seen in the lower leg
- Cellulitis: inflammation of the soft tissues

Q: *What activities can be helpful in muscle recovery for the legs?*

A: Swimming is a wonderful activity to help the body recover from excessive exercise or injury. Water running and swimming are both helpful—in the water, the body exercises in a basically gravity-free environment, which promotes circulation and increases strength without the pounding of the joints. Hot-and-cold contrast applications are valuable for tendon pain due to overexertion or injury. Start with cold (two minutes), then heat (one minute), then cold again (two minutes), and so on; always start and end with cold. Massage therapy and stretching are also important for improving circulation during recovery.

Prevention Is the Key

- Warm up before exercise and cool down afterward.
- Keep the body well hydrated.
- Use properly fitted sports equipment, particularly shoes.
- Maintain a balance of muscle strength.

ANKLE PAIN

Ankle pain may be the result of ankle twisting, poor biomechanics (body movement), or direct trauma to the muscles, tendons, and ligaments. Conditions associated with ankle pain include:

- Ankle sprain: overstretching or tearing of ligaments in the ankle joint
  - Mild or first-degree sprain: a minimal tear or stretch of the ligaments, which connect bone to bone

- Moderate or second-degree sprain: a partial tear of the ligament (weight bearing may be difficult)
- Severe or third-degree sprain: a complete tear of a ligament; could also be accompanied by a fracture

• Ankle strain: inflammation of the tendons of the ankle

Stretching, exercises to strengthen the ankle, and massage can all help alleviate pain in the ankle.

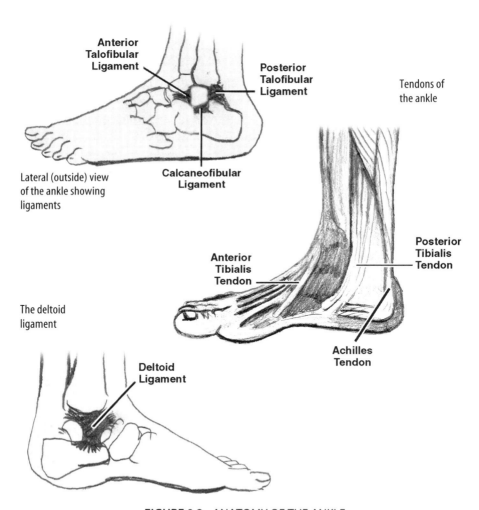

FIGURE 9.2. ANATOMY OF THE ANKLE

ANKLE PAIN OVERVIEW	
Signs and Symptoms	**Causes**
• Swelling	• Violent, twisting motion
• Pain and point tenderness	• Rolling of the ankle
• Deformity	• Direct trauma or blow
• Discoloration	• Stress on the joint itself due to poor biomechanics (body movement)
• Loss of function (including difficulty bearing weight)	
	• Poor arch formation in foot (flat or high arches)

Recipe for a Healthy Ankle

1. Start each day by stretching the hamstrings, feet, and lower-leg muscles to get them warmed up and ready for activity; hold each stretch for two seconds only, and repeat eight to ten times. Always return to the starting position before the next repetition and exhale your breath on the stretch phase. Also stretch before and after activity at other times of day.

2. Strengthening exercises can be done two to three times weekly, with one day of rest in between. Always stretch before you strengthen.

3. Perform RICHES: rest, ice, compression, heat, elevation, and support (see Chapter 3).

4. Massage with ice or apply ice bags or packs two to four times daily for ten minutes each time (especially after exercise).

5. Supportive bracing or wrapping may be helpful during recovery. For severe ankle sprains, crutches may be necessary to avoid placing weight on the ankle.

6. Massage therapy, which is helpful for flushing out the swelling, can be applied one to two times daily. For severe strains, avoid deep massage techniques.

7. When returning to exercise or activity, stretch and warm up first. Gradually increase exercise levels as symptoms or pain begin to dissipate. Always cool down properly, remember to stretch, and apply ice when finished.

8. Maintain a proper diet and hydration for recovery (see Chapter 2).

Stretches for the Ankle

A number of stretches have proven effective in promoting flexibility and alleviating ankle pain.

Plantar Flexion Stretch

While seated, flex the left knee and place the ankle across the knee of the opposite leg. Place your right hand on top of the foot and point the foot, gently assisting

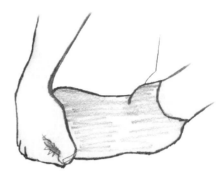

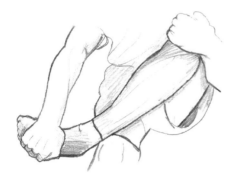

with your hand. This will stretch the shin muscle. Exhale on the stretch phase and hold for two seconds, then return to the starting position. Repeat eight to ten times. Then, perform the same stretch with the right leg.

Calf Stretch

Place a rope around the ball of your right foot, and sit on the floor with your leg extended (the knee should be straight). The opposite leg should be bent to help ease any low-back or hamstring discomfort. Bring the top of your right foot toward your chest, using the rope to assist. Avoid leaning

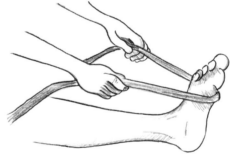

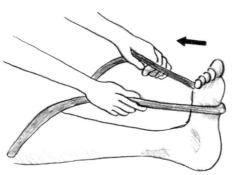

back while assisting yourself during the stretch phase. Maintain a 90-degree angle at the hip, using your arms only to assist yourself with the rope. Exhale on the stretch phase and hold for two seconds, then return to the starting position. Repeat eight to ten times. Then, repeat the stretch with the left leg.

Soleus Stretch

Sit on the floor with your knee flexed and your foot resting on the floor. Lift the foot toward your chest while keeping the heel on the floor. Assist the

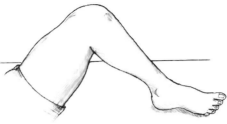

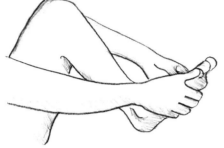

stretch with your hands under the ball of the foot (may use a rope, if necessary). Exhale on the stretch phase and hold for two seconds, then return to the starting position. Repeat eight to ten times. Then, perform the stretch with the other foot.

Achilles Tendon Stretch

Sit on the floor and flex one knee, bringing your heel as close as possible to your buttocks. Flex your forefoot and toes toward your chest, assisting with your hands under the ball of the foot (may use a rope, if necessary). Exhale on the stretch phase and hold for two seconds, then return to the starting position. Repeat eight to ten times. Then, perform the stretch with the other foot.

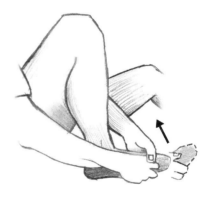

Extension of Toes

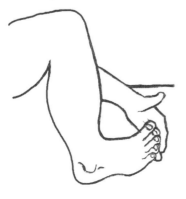

While seated, flex one knee and gently bring your heel toward your buttocks. Extend each toe back as far as possible, assisting with your hand. Exhale on the stretch phase and hold for two seconds, then return to the starting position. Repeat eight to ten times. Then, perform the stretch with the other foot. (Extending the toes also stretches the arch of the foot.)

Ankle Inversion and Eversion Stretch

While seated, wrap a rope around the ball of your foot. Turn the ankle inward and flex your toes and foot toward your chest, gently assisting with the rope. Exhale on the stretch phase and hold for two seconds, then return to

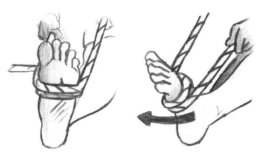

the starting position. Repeat eight to ten times. Then, turn the ankle outward, again flexing the foot and assisting the stretch with the rope. Exhale on the stretch phase and hold for two seconds, then return to the starting position. Repeat eight to ten times. Perform the same stretch on the other foot.

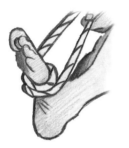 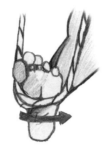

Exercises for the Ankle

The following exercises will help you condition your ankle muscles and recover from injury.

Toe Scrunches

Place a towel on the floor with a small weight placed on top at one end of the towel. Grasp the towel with your toes, pulling the weight toward your heel. You

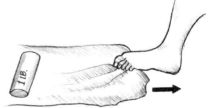

may need to dampen your toes for a better grip. When finished, straighten the towel and repeat ten to fifteen times. Then, perform the exercise with the other foot.

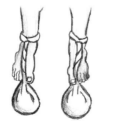 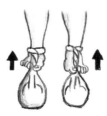

Dorsiflexion Exercise I

Place a small weight in a tube sock (or pillowcase) and tie the end of the sock around your ankle, feeding it between the big toe and second toe. Tie another weighted sock around your other ankle. Sit on an elevated platform, such as a tall table, so that the feet do not touch the floor and the weighted tube socks just skim the surface of the floor. Then, lift up ankles and feet. Return to the starting position and repeat fifteen times. Add more weight if necessary.

Dorsiflexion Exercise II

Follow the instructions for dorsiflexion exercise I above, with the following variation: Turn your ankles outward while lifting your ankles and feet upward. Repeat fifteen times. Add more weight if necessary.

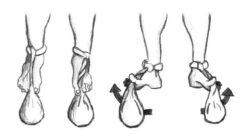

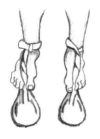
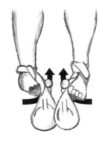

Dorsiflexion Exercise III

Follow the instructions for dorsiflexion exercise I above, with the following variation: Turn your ankles inward while lifting your ankles and feet upward. Repeat fifteen times. Add more weight if necessary.

Calf Raises

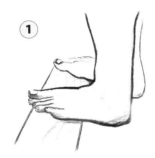

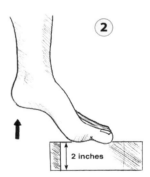

Place the ball of the foot and the toes on a two-inch-high board. Heels should rest on the floor. Hold on to the wall or a chair for support and raise up onto your toes. To isolate the inner and outer calf muscles, turn your toes inward and raise up for ten repetitions, then turn your toes outward and raise up for ten repetitions. Exhale on the work phase.

2 inches

Fun Fact

Have you ever wondered why you most often roll your ankle and foot to the inside rather than to the outside? Rolling your ankle to the outside, which injures the inside of your ankle, is uncommon due to the anatomical bone structures of the lower leg and the strength of the deltoid ligament, located underneath the "knobby prominence" on the inside of your ankle.

Massage Techniques for the Ankle

These massage techniques can relieve muscle spasm and pain, increase circulation, and promote the healing of ankle injuries.

Fanning of the Ankle (Assisted Massage)

The massage assistant places the heel in one palm to stabilize the foot. With the other hand, he or she uses the palm surface of his or her hand to gently massage around the ankle joint, using circular motions. The mas-

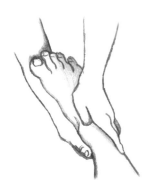

sage assistant can also gently glide up the shin muscle (not the shin bone) for a finishing stroke. Repeat as necessary.

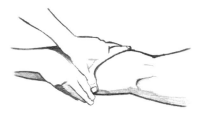

Top-of-Ankle Assisted Massage

The massage assistant places one hand gently on the top of the foot. With the other hand, he or she uses the palm surface of his or her hand to massage the shin muscle (not the bone). The massage assistant should simultaneously glide one hand up the shin while pointing the foot and toes down with the other hand (using gentle pressure). For severe ankle sprains, avoid pointing the toes and foot downward. Repeat as necessary.

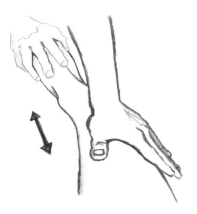

When to Call the Doctor

- If you experience numbness or tingling

- If there is any deformity

- If you chronically suffer from cold feet

- If there is severe swelling or you are unable to walk

Questions and Answers

Q: *Why do ankle sprains recur so easily?*

A: Ankle sprains may happen again for several reasons, including:

A return to activity before complete recovery

Laxity (looseness) in the ankle ligaments due to chronic overstretching or tearing

Lack of proper rehabilitation, treatment, stretching, and strengthening of ligaments and surrounding soft tissues that support the ankle

Wearing improper shoes (for example, athletic shoes that don't provide enough ankle support)

Failure to get a proper diagnosis of the ankle injury in the first place

---

Prevention is the Key

- Warm up before exercise and cool down afterward.
- Use properly fitted sports equipment, including shoes.
- Maintain a balance of muscle strength.
- Avoid running on rough, uneven surfaces.

FOOT PAIN

Timmy was born with "club feet": pigeon-toed, minimum arch support, and bowed-out legs. So began a long odyssey of braces, casts, and corrective shoes to try and fix the deformity. He made great progress, but at the age of ten Timmy started to experience a lot of discomfort in his lower back and feet, no doubt due to the growth spurts he was now going through. It looked as though surgery was the most viable option. His parents decided to research other alternatives and try to avoid surgery. After a couple of recommendations, Timmy's parents brought him to see me (Kim).

Three times a week, I worked with Timmy on a series of stretches and exercises to increase flexibility and strength in the entire lower body, including all muscles, ligaments, and tendons. Immediately, the range of motion improved in his hips, allowing him to walk with a more normal gait. This dramatically improved the low-back pain he was experiencing. Gradually, the range of motion in his feet also began to improve. I also recommended orthotic shoe inserts for better support. He stuck with the program and made great progress over the next two years. Today, Timmy runs, rides his bike, and plays soccer and lacrosse just like all the other kids his age. Most important, he learned the importance of stretching at an early age and how it can help alleviate pain and promote recovery.

Foot pain may result from placing too much stress on the heel bone, overuse or overexertion of the plantar muscles, or direct trauma to both the bone and muscle. Conditions associated with foot pain include:

- Bruise of the heel bone: can occur while walking, running, or jumping on hard surfaces

- Heel spur: a bony growth on the underside of the heel bone, which could irritate the muscles and ligaments on the bottom of the foot

- Plantar fasciitis: inflammation of the muscle that runs along the bottom of the foot from the heel bone to the ball of the foot

Running or any contact sport may lead to foot injuries. Other factors in foot pain may include being overweight or inactive, as well as lacking flexibility—particularly, having tight calves and hamstrings.

Stretching, exercises to strengthen the muscles supporting the foot, and massage can all help alleviate foot pain.

FOOT PAIN OVERVIEW

Signs and Symptoms	*Causes*
• Sharp pain on the bottom of the heel	• Previous foot, ankle, or heel injury
• Pain when stepping out of bed in the morning	• Tight muscles on the bottom of the foot or in the calf
• Point tenderness of the heel bone	• Excessive weight-bearing activity from obesity
• Loss of strength	• Over-pronation of the foot (heel moves outward, ankle moves inward)
	• Excessive running or jogging
	• Weakness in the bottom of the foot
	• Aggravation from prolonged weight bearing and walking

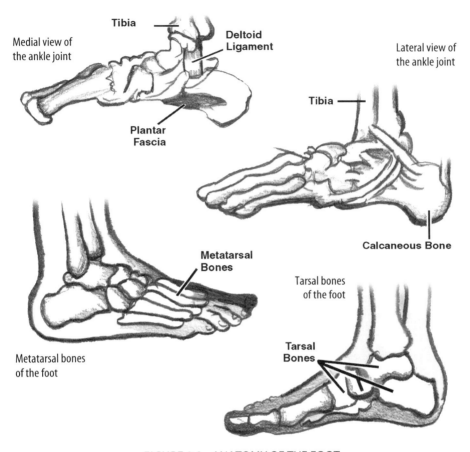

Tibia

Deltoid Ligament

Medial view of the ankle joint

Lateral view of the ankle joint

Tibia

Plantar Fascia

Calcaneous Bone

Metatarsal Bones

Tarsal bones of the foot

Tarsal Bones

Metatarsal bones of the foot

FIGURE 9.3. ANATOMY OF THE FOOT

Recipe for a Healthy Foot

1. Stretch the foot, calf, and hamstring muscles one to two times daily (especially before and after exercise). Hold each stretch for two seconds and return to the starting position before the next repetition. Repeat eight to ten times; exhale on the stretch phase.

2. Perform RICHES: rest, ice, compression, heat, elevation, and support (see Chapter 3).

3. Massage with ice two to four times daily for ten minutes each time; always keep ice in contact with the skin, moving ice in a circular motion. You can also roll your foot on a soda bottle filled with frozen water.

4. Do strengthening exercises two to three times weekly, with one day of rest in between. Always stretch before you strengthen. Icing after strengthening is also helpful.

5. Self-massage can be applied one to two times daily.

6. When returning to exercise, warm up and stretch first. Gradually increase your exercise level as your symptoms improve. Cool down properly, followed by stretching and icing.

7. Wear supportive shoes.

8. Maintain a proper diet and hydration for recovery (see Chapter 2).

Stretches for the Foot

A number of stretches have proven effective in promoting flexibility and alleviating foot pain.

Calf Stretch

Place a rope around the ball of your right foot, and sit on the floor with your leg extended (the knee should be straight). The opposite leg should be bent to help ease any low-back or hamstring discomfort. Bring the top of the right foot toward your chest, using the rope to assist. Avoid lean-

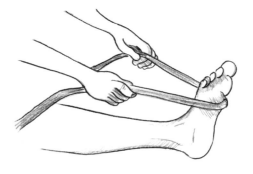

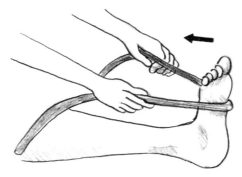

ing back while assisting yourself during the stretch phase. Maintain a 90-degree angle at the hip, using your arms only to assist yourself with the rope. Exhale on the stretch phase and hold for two seconds, then return to the starting position. Repeat eight to ten times. Then, repeat the stretch with the left leg.

Soleus Stretch

Sit on the floor with your knee flexed and your foot resting on the floor. Lift the foot toward your chest while keeping the heel on the floor. Assist the

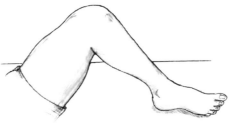

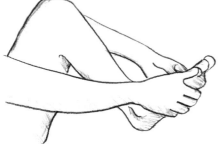

stretch with your hands under the ball of the foot (may use a rope, if necessary). Exhale on the stretch phase and hold for two seconds, then return to the starting position. Repeat eight to ten times. Then, perform the stretch with the other foot.

Achilles Tendon Stretch

Sit on the floor and flex one knee, bringing your heel as close as possible to your buttocks. Flex your forefoot and toes toward your chest, assisting with your hands under the ball of the foot (may use a rope, if necessary). Exhale on the stretch phase and hold for two seconds, then return to the starting position. Repeat eight to ten times. Then, perform the stretch with the other foot.

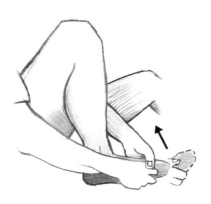

Extension of Toes

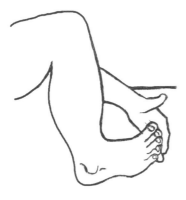

While seated, flex one knee and gently bring your heel toward your buttocks. Extend each toe back as far as possible, assisting with your hand. Exhale on the stretch phase and hold for two seconds, then return to the starting position. Repeat eight to ten times. Then, perform the stretch with the other foot. (Extending the toes also stretches the arch of the foot.)

Ankle Inversion and Eversion Stretch

While seated, wrap a rope around the ball of your foot. Turn the ankle inward and flex your toes and foot toward your chest, gently assisting with the rope. Exhale on the stretch phase and hold for two seconds, then return to

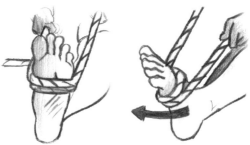

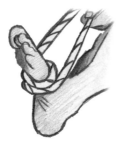
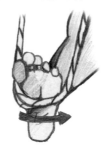

the starting position. Repeat eight to ten times, then turn the ankle outward, again flexing the foot and assisting the stretch with the rope. Exhale on the stretch phase and hold for two seconds, then return to the starting position. Repeat eight to ten times. Perform the same stretch on the other foot.

Exercises for the Foot

The following exercises will help you condition your foot muscles and recover from injury.

Toe Scrunches

Place a towel on the floor with a small weight placed on top at one end of the towel. Grasp the towel with your toes, pulling the weight toward your heel. You

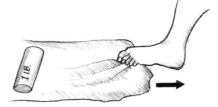

may need to dampen your toes for a better grip. When finished, straighten the towel and repeat ten to fifteen times. Then, perform the exercise with the other foot.

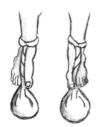
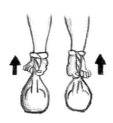

Dorsiflexion Exercise I

Place a small weight in a tube sock (or pillowcase) and tie the end of the sock around your ankle, feeding it between the big toe and second toe. Tie another weighted sock around your other ankle. Sit on an elevated platform, such

as a tall table, so that the feet do not touch the floor and the weighted tube socks just skim the surface of the floor. Then, lift up ankles and feet. Return to the starting position and repeat fifteen times. Add more weight if necessary.

Dorsiflexion Exercise II

Follow the instructions for dorsiflexion exercise I above, with the following variation: Turn your ankles outward while lifting your ankles and feet upward. Repeat fifteen times. Add more weight if necessary.

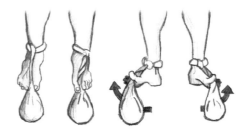

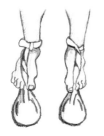 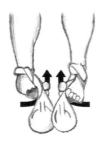

Dorsiflexion Exercise III

Follow the instructions for dorsiflexion exercise I above, with the following variation: Turn your ankles inward while lifting your ankles and feet upward. Repeat fifteen times. Add more weight if necessary.

Calf Raises

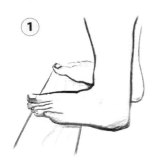

Place the ball of the foot and the toes on a two-inch-high board. Heels should rest on the floor. Hold on to the wall or a chair for support and raise up onto your toes. To isolate the inner and outer calf muscles, turn your toes inward and raise up for ten repetitions, then turn your toes outward and raise up for ten repetitions. Exhale on the work phase.

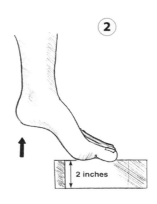

2 inches

Massage Techniques for the Foot

These massage techniques can relieve muscle spasm and pain, increase circulation, and promote the healing of foot injuries.

Assisted Foot Massage

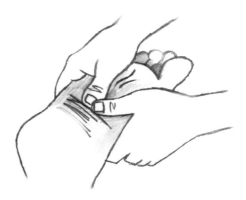

Lie on your stomach with your knee flexed and the bottom of your foot facing the ceiling. The massage assistant places both thumbs along the bottom of the foot and glides along the surface. He or she massages the entire foot and uses circular friction with his or her thumbs at the heel, if needed. Repeat as necessary.

Fanning of the Ankle (Assisted Massage)

The massage assistant places the heel in one palm to stabilize the foot. With the other hand, he or she uses the palm surface of his or her hand to gently massage around the ankle joint, using circular motions. The mas-

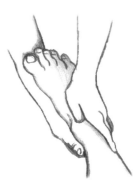

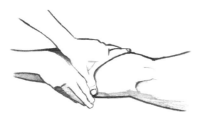

sage assistant can also gently glide up the shin muscle (not the shin bone) for a finishing stroke. Repeat as necessary.

When to Call the Doctor

- If pain persists despite treatment
- If you experience numbness or tingling
- If there is severe swelling or you are unable to walk

Questions and Answers

Q: *Can I overstretch my calf and foot muscles and make my condition worse?*

A: It is possible to overstretch an area if the applied stretch is incorrect. Follow the protocol for stretching the calves and feet. If you continue to be sore after stretching, then that would be an indication that you are stretching too aggressively. Remember to hold stretches for two seconds only, then return to the starting position; repeat eight to ten times.

Q: *Do I need a rope to help me stretch or can I use my arms?*

A: Using your arms and hands can sometimes stress other areas of the body, taking away your full concentration from the stretch. Using a rope is the most effective way to assist yourself in stretching. Some people prefer a long towel rolled up or a bathrobe tie, both of which are fine but sometimes tend to be a bit short in length. A seven-foot piece of rope works best.

Q: *Should I ice before stretching?*

A: Icing sore areas before stretching is effective and helpful. Although not required, icing will cool down the area while flushing away inflammation in the foot or heel. Follow icing with gentle stretching to help promote a fresh blood supply to the area, assisting in the healing cycle.

Prevention Is the Key

- Start each day with gentle stretches to prepare your body for movement and activity.

- Drink plenty of water: the muscles that drive body movements are 75 percent water.

- End each day with a cooling-down process: stretch lightly to relax fatigued muscles, as it will help them circulate fresh oxygenated blood throughout your body. Also, relax your mind by practicing deep breathing and meditation.

- Affirmation: be appreciative and thankful for what the day has brought to you.

Chapter 10

If Your Pain Doesn't Go Away

We have taken you through an extensive journey of discovery, pain self-identification, and action steps to help you with your condition. But what do you do if your pain does not go away? The first thing to remember is, don't give up. Your condition may cause pain, frustration, and even depression, but it is crucial to your recovery that you be persistent in seeking a solution and have a positive approach to achieving a better quality of life. Throughout this book, we have shown that a positive mental attitude works, with many examples of people who have overcome or managed their pain with a proactive approach.

In this chapter, we include answers to some additional healthcare questions to help you continue on your journey to better health:

- When should I see a doctor?

- What questions are appropriate to ask my doctor?

- How do I keep the attention of my doctor?

- To what extent do I "stick to my guns" and avoid being put off by my doctor?

WHEN SHOULD I SEE A DOCTOR?
In the event of a critical, life-threatening injury or illness, always activate the emergency medical system (EMS) by calling 911. How do you know if the situation is critical? If the victim does not have an open airway, is not breathing, is bleeding profusely, or if circulation has ceased, it is an emergency. Activating EMS is the most important action step in an emergency situation. We recommend that you educate yourself further by learning cardiopulmonary resuscitation (CPR) and first aid through the American Red Cross or the American Heart Association.

In the case of a noncritical injury or illness, it is always better to err on the side of caution. In other words, have a doctor or other healthcare practitioner examine and diagnose your condition early rather than leave yourself "wondering" if something is wrong, searching for answers in books or on the Internet, and ultimately delaying medical care. Even if you can't afford a doctor's visit, you can still be evaluated at a local public hospital or public health department.

Here are some other suggestions about when to see the doctor:

- If you have persistent pain, either sharp or dull, that does not go away despite taking all the appropriate action steps that are detailed in this book. This could be a sign of a chronic illness such as arthritis.

- If you have an onset of pain for no apparent reason; for example, a sudden pain in your lower right abdomen could be appendicitis.

- If you feel numbness or tingling around an injured area or other region; for example, you may have no feeling or sensation in your fingers due to a hand or wrist injury.

- If bleeding is not easily controlled or you have skin discoloration; for example, a severe cut that will not stop bleeding despite first-aid steps, including direct pressure and elevation.

- If there is deformity, such as a broken bone that creates a lump or bump at the injured site.

- If there are signs of infection: redness around the injury, swelling, heat, and pain.

- If there is significant swelling, such as puffiness around a sprained ankle.

- If you experience loss of function, range of motion, or weight-bearing ability; that is, if you are unable to move a body part, lack flexibility, experience chronic joint pain, limp, or can't walk.

- If you have a fever, prolonged vomiting or diarrhea, elevated temperature, or upset stomach.

- If you experience other unusual signs or symptoms: rash, changes in the wound's appearance, rapid changes in weight, or constant fatigue.

What Are the Appropriate Questions to Ask My Doctor?

Do not be afraid to ask questions about your condition. Follow these guidelines when asking questions to get the answers you need from your physician:

- Ask for clarification in layperson's terms if you do not understand the medical terminology being used; for example, "Could you explain osteochondritis dissecans (OCD) of the knee in simple terms?"

- Ask specific questions related to your condition, such as "Is there a cure for my tendinitis?"

- Ask if additional diagnostic test(s)—MRI (magnetic resonance imaging), x-ray, computed tomography (CT) scan, and so on—would be appropriate for your condition.

- Ask questions related to your short-term and long-term outlook or prognosis: "How many days/weeks will it take for my sprained ankle to heal?" (short-term prognosis); "Will I be referred to a physical therapist following my surgery?" (long-term prognosis).

- Ask about the side effects or risks related to your treatment or therapy regimen, including surgery.

- Ask for helpful resources for more information about your condition.

- Ask about approximate costs of treatments and procedures, if this is a concern for you.

- Ask if there is an effective generic alternative that may be less expensive than the prescribed brand-name drug. Also, inquire if your physician has any free samples of medications that would be appropriate in treating your condition.

- Be respectful when asking questions of your doctor, even if you disagree with him or her; for example, "Doctor, with all due respect, I disagree with your diagnosis. What other options are available for me?"

- Ask if the addition of other healthcare providers would be appropriate in managing your condition; for example, "Would a chiropractor, massage therapist, or physical therapist be beneficial for my whiplash?"

- Ask about rehabilitation or other therapies related to your condition and reemphasize that you will be proactive as a patient; for example, "Would referral to a certified hand therapist (CHT) aid in my recovery? I promise to be accountable for my hand injury and will comply with all instructions for rehabilitation."

- Ask about the necessity for follow-up appointments or referral to other healthcare professionals or specialists.

- Ask if there are any support groups or other patients that you could interact with for additional help.

How Do I Keep the Attention of My Doctor?

In today's medical world, physicians and other healthcare providers are required to see more patients in a shorter amount of time. This means that your healthcare professional may have only a brief amount of time to interact with you, based on the severity of your injury or illness. The key in this situation is to maximize the time you have with your doctor and use it efficiently.

Here are some suggestions for keeping your doctor's attention:

• Interact with the physician and let them know when something hurts—don't be shy or clam up.

• Don't force the physician to be a detective—be honest and thorough about your condition and symptoms.

• Give the doctor specific feedback related to your condition; for example, "The bottom of my foot hurts the most in the morning when I am getting out of bed."

• Be respectful even if you disagree with your doctor.

• Explain that you will be proactive, positive, and accountable as a patient.

• Don't bring in an extensive "laundry list" of questions unless invited to do so by the physician—you should ask questions covered in the previous section, but use common sense.

• Be courteous, interactive, and smile or laugh during your office visit.

To What Extent Do I "Stick to My Guns" and Avoid Being Put Off by My Doctor?

Remember that doctors are human beings. They have the same emotions and feelings that you do. Keep in mind that your doctor may be having a "bad day" or suffering from lack of sleep. Try to check the credentials of your provider in advance and keep in mind that most healthcare professionals want to work with you in treating your condition.

Here are some suggestions to avoid being put off by your doctor:

• Keep your comments as positive as possible; for example, "How can I assist you in finding another, alternative treatment for my condition?"

• Make eye contact, speak clearly, and smile during your interaction with a healthcare professional.

• If possible, do research about your condition in advance of your visit to the doctor.

- Ask for a recheck or follow-up visits; for example, "Could I return to your office in two weeks for a recheck of my condition?"

- If you are still not clear about your condition after asking questions, ask if there is another qualified person available to discuss your condition.

- Again, be polite even if you disagree with your doctor; for example, "Doctor, with all due respect, I do not agree with your diagnosis. Could this condition be the result of something else?"

- If appropriate, let your doctor know that you will be seeking another opinion (especially for surgery).

- Keep an accurate medical file on your condition, such as a chronological file of your doctor's appointments, bills, and insurance policy. Also, ask for copies of test results (MRIs, blood tests, x-rays) and other related information.

- Make appointments for follow-ups and referrals in person, if possible—this may help avoid confusion.

- Call early in the day for refills and other appointments—give your provider as much time as possible to respond. Leave clear and accurate messages, including your name, phone number, and pharmacy.

- Make sure you understand the directions about taking your medications, dosages, and uses (how much medicine to take and exactly when). Also, ask about taking your medication with or without food.

- Be appreciative of your doctor's care—thank your doctor and other healthcare providers for their time or send a thank-you card, if appropriate.

YOUR JOURNEY TO BETTER HEALTH AND HAPPINESS

Your pain may continue despite all the suggestions listed in this book, but we suggest that you persist in your journey toward better health. Remember, your health is one of your most important assets.

Seek out other healing modalities and healthcare providers to assist you in achieving a better quality of life. Although these therapies and providers are not covered in this book, they may be a viable solution for your condition: chronic-pain clinics, proven alternative therapies, physiatrists, osteopaths, homeopaths, and acupuncturists. When choosing any healthcare professional, check credentials, licenses, and talk to other patients, if necessary.

We hope that we have helped you understand, recognize, and alleviate your pain. Keep in mind that your positive mental attitude and willingness to be proactive in your recovery are the key elements to better living. Remember that your body is connected from head to toe through the mind, body, and soul. Adopt healthy habits and get on the road to recovery today.

Good luck in the rest of your journey and live well!

Appendix

Pain-Related Websites

Refer to Chapter 2, pages 20–21, for guidance on using health-related websites.

Active Isolated Stretching (Mattes Method): www.stretchingusa.com

American Academy of Orthopaedic Surgeons: www.aaos.org

American Academy of Pain Management: www.aapainmanage.org

American Chronic Pain Association: www.theacpa.org

American Heart Association: www.americanheart.org

American Holistic Medical Association: www.holisticmedicine.org

American Pain Foundation: www.painfoundation.org

American Pain Society: www.ampainsoc.org

American Podiatric Medical Association: www.apma.org

American Stroke Association: www.strokeassociation.org

Arthritis Foundation: www.arthritis.org

Chronic Fatigue and Immune Dysfunction Syndrome Association of America: www.cfids.org

ErgAerobics Inc. (ergonomic aerobics): www.ergaerobics.com

Fibromyalgia Network: www.fmnetnews.com

The Lupus Foundation of America: www.lupus.org

Muscular Dystrophy Association: www.mdausa.org

The National Foundation for the Treatment of Pain: www.paincare.org

National Headache Foundation: www.headaches.org

National Institute of Environmental Health Sciences: www.niehs.nih.gov

National Institutes of Health: www.nih.gov

National Library of Medicine (NLM): www.nlm.nih.gov

National Multiple Sclerosis Society: www.nmss.org

National Osteoporosis Foundation: www.nof.org

National Sleep Foundation: www.sleepfoundation.org

Occupational Safety and Health Administration (OSHA): www.osha.gov

T'ai Chi: www.scheele.org/lee/taichi.html

WebMD: www.webmd.com

Glossary

Abduction. movement away from the midline of the body.

Acute injury. condition with sudden onset and short duration.

Adduction. movement toward the midline of the body.

Anterior. in front of or before.

Anxiety. a feeling of uncertainty or apprehension.

Apophysis. bony outgrowth to which muscles attach.

Atrophy. wasting away or decrease in the size of tissue.

Bursitis. inflammation of the bursa, which is a fluid-filled sac; provides protection and helps reduce friction between bony prominences.

Cardiorespiratory endurance. ability to sustain physical exertion over an extended period of time.

Chiropractor. one who practices a method for restoring normal health by adjusting the segments of the spinal column.

Chondromalacia. abnormal softening of the cartilage, usually in the knee.

Chronic injury. condition with long onset and long duration.

Circumduct. act of moving a limb in a circular manner.

Contrast applications. alternating applications of ice and heat at varying time intervals depending on the injury, always ending with ice treatment.

Degree of injury. first—mild; second—moderate; and third—severe.

Diagnosis. identification of a specific condition.

Distal. farthest from the midline or center of the body.

Dorsiflexion. bending toes toward the body.

Edema. swelling as a result of fluid in connective tissue.

Elevation. to raise a part of the body above the level of the heart.

Endurance. the body's ability to sustain exertion over time.

Epicondylitis. inflammation on the medial (inner) or lateral (outer) part of the elbow.

Extension. to straighten or move away from the midline.

Fascia. fibrous membrane that covers and supports muscles.

Fasciitis. inflammation of the fascia.

Flexibility. the amount of range of motion at a joint.

Flexion. bending or flexing.

Gait. manner or style of walking.

Gluteal. pertaining to the buttocks or the muscles that form the buttocks.

Hamstring muscles. group of three muscles on the back of the thigh; responsible for knee flexion.

Heat therapy. application of heat in the form of packs, whirlpool, paraffin, or pads.

Hematoma. a mass of blood that forms as a result of a broken blood vessel.

Homeostasis. maintenance of a steady state.

Ice therapy. application of ice in the form of bags, packs, cups, slush bucket, or whirlpool.

Iliotibial band syndrome (ITBS). "runner's knee" or inflammation of the iliotibial band.

Injury. act that hurts or damages.

Joint capsule. saclike structure that surrounds the ends of the bones.

Kyphosis. abnormal curvature of the thoracic spine.

Lordosis. abnormal curvature of the lumbar vertebrae.

Lumbar. lower region of the back.

Massage. touching of the skin to promote healing; various forms include effleurage, petrissage, tapotement, and friction.

Metatarsalgia. inflammation to the metatarsals of the foot, including the ball of the foot.

Myositis. inflammation of the muscles.

Nerve entrapment. nerve compressed between bones or soft tissues.

Neuritis. inflammation of a nerve.

Obesity. excessive amount of body fat.

Orthopedic surgeon. one who corrects deformities of the musculoskeletal system.

Orthotic. an appliance or apparatus, such as a brace or splint, used to support, align, prevent, or correct deformities or to improve function.

Osteoarthritis. chronic disease involving joints in which there is destruction of articular cartilage and bony overgrowth.

Osteochondritis dissecans. fragments of cartilage and underlying bone detached from the articular surface.

Osteoporosis. condition characterized by a decrease in bone density.

Podiatrist. practitioner who specializes in the study and care of the foot.

Point tenderness. pain produced in a specific area when touched.

Posterior. toward the back or rear.

Prognosis. prediction as to the probable outcome of an injury or illness.

Quadriceps muscles. group of four muscles on the front of the thigh responsible for knee extension.

Radiate. to diverge or emerge from a central point.

Referred pain. pain that occurs at a site other than the point of origin.

RICHES. rest, ice, compression, heat, elevation, and support.

Scoliosis. lateral curvature of the spine.

Sign. objective evidence of an abnormal situation within the body.

Stress. positive or negative forces that can disrupt the body's equilibrium.

Symptom. subjective evidence that indicates injury or illness.

Tendinitis. inflammation of a tendon.

Trauma. wound or injury usually due to direct contact.

Trigger points. small hyperirritable areas within a muscle.

Vertebrae. Thirty-three bones in the spine that protect the cord and serve as a place for soft tissue attachments.

Vitamin. an organic compound essential in small quantities for normal function.

Weakness. lack of strength.

X-ray. radiograph used to capture images of bones and cavities.

Yoga. discipline that focuses on the body's musculature, posture, breathing, and consciousness.

References

Ballard, Jim. *Mind Like Water: Keeping Your Balance in a Chaotic World*. Hoboken, NJ: John Wiley & Sons, 2002.

Bodian, Stephan. *Meditation for Dummies*. New York: Hungry Minds, 1999.

Canfield, Jack, and Mark Victor Hansen. *Dare to Win*. New York: Berkley Publishing Group, 1994.

Canfield, Jack, Mark Victor Hansen, and Les Hewitt. *The Power of Focus: How to Hit Your Business, Personal and Financial Targets with Absolute Certainty*. Deerfield Beach, FL: Health Communications, 2000.

Capellini, Steve, and Michel Van Welden. *Massage for Dummies*. New York: Hungry Minds, 1999.

Chaitow, Leon. *Conquer Pain the Natural Way*. San Francisco: Chronicle Books, 2002.

Fishman, Scott, and Lisa Berger. *The War on Pain*. New York: HarperCollins Publishers, 2001.

Harrell, Keith. *Attitude Is Everything: 10 Life-Changing Steps to Turning Attitude Into Action*. New York: Harper Business, 2003.

Harrison, Eric. *Teach Yourself to Meditate in 10 Simple Lessons*. Berkeley, CA: Ulysses Press, 2001.

Mattes, Aaron. *Specific Stretching for Everyone*. Sarasota, FL: Aaron Mattes Therapy, 1995.

Richardson, Cheryl. *Take Time for Your Life: A Personal Coach's Seven-Step Program for Creating the Life You Want*. New York: Broadway Books, 1998.

Sarno, John. *Healing Back Pain*. New York: Warner Books, 1991.

Schlosberg, Suzanne, and Liz Neporent. *Fitness for Dummies*. New York: Hungry Minds, 2000.

Sharkey, Brian. *Fitness and Health*. 5th ed. Champaign, IL: Human Kinetics, 2002.

Sharp, Timothy. *The Good Sleep Guide: 10 Steps to Better Sleep and How to Break the Worry Cycle*. Berkeley, CA: Frog Ltd., 2001.

Siegel, Bernie S., M.D. *Love, Medicine, and Miracles*. New York: Perennial, 1990.

U.S. Consumer Products Safety Commission, Directorate for Epidemiology. "National Electronic Injury Surveillance System (NEISS)." Washington, DC: National Injury Information Clearinghouse, 2004. Accessed via the Internet at www.cpsc.gov/library/neiss.html.

Wolinsky, Howard, and Judi Wolinsky. *Healthcare Online for Dummies*. New York: Hungry Minds, 2001.

Index

About the Authors

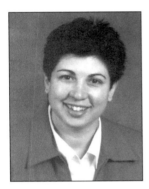

Angela Sehgal, Ed.D., A.T.C./L., holds a doctorate degree in Educational Leadership and Policy Studies from Florida State University (FSU) in Tallahassee, Florida. She earned her M.S. degree in Athletic Administration from FSU and her B.A. from Anderson University in Anderson, Indiana.

Since 1988, Dr. Sehgal has been an athletic trainer, certified by the National Athletic Trainers' Association Board of Certification (NATABOC) and licensed as a certified athletic trainer by the state of Florida. She served as an assistant athletic trainer in the FSU Athletic Department from 1991 to 2001. She is now a full-time faculty member of the FSU Nutrition, Food, and Exercise Sciences Department, serving as the curriculum coordinator for the athletic-training/sports-medicine education program.

Dr. Sehgal enjoys spending time with her family, friends, and dogs and continually strives to lower her golf score.

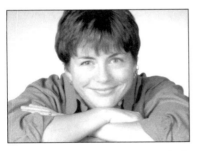

Kim Ortloff, L.M.T., has a degree from Florida State University (FSU) in exercise physiology. She is a graduate of the CORE Institute of Massage Therapy and a licensed massage therapist in Tallahassee, Florida, where she has owned and operated a massage therapy and flexibility clinic for the past ten years. Kim continues to study with Aaron Mattes, kinesiologist and founder of the Mattes Method of Active Isolated Stretching (AIS), at his rehabilitative facility in Sarasota, Florida. She has assisted Mattes in teaching AIS nationwide to massage therapists, physical therapists, chiropractors, and athletic trainers.

Kim has supported athletes at national and international events. She worked at the 1996 Summer Olympics in the sports massage clinic and has served as a team therapist for both FSU men's and women's swim teams. In 1999, she served as the team therapist for Zimbabwe at the World Track-and-Field Championship in Seville, Spain. In 2003, Kim served as team therapist for FSU's track team at NCAA national championships. She has been featured as a guest lecturer at FSU, where she works closely with the athletic department. Kim is currently working with National Football League players.

Kim lives in Tallahassee with her husband, John, and their four cats and three dogs. She teaches locally about motivation and goal setting as well as the promotion and application of health and wellness.

Please visit

http://www.whereithurtsandwhy.com

*for more information on
pain-related topics.*